INTO
SANITY

INTO SANITY

ESSAYS ABOUT
MENTAL HEALTH, MENTAL ILLNESS,
AND LIVING IN BETWEEN

A TALKING WRITING ANTHOLOGY

EDITED BY MARTHA NICHOLS
PREFACE BY MARK VONNEGUT

Talking Writing Books
Cambridge, Massachusetts

Into Sanity: Essays About Mental Health, Mental Illness, and Living in Between is a work of nonfiction. In some essays, names and identifying details have been changed.

Copyright © 2019 by Talking Writing, Inc. All Rights Reserved.

The following essays have previously been published in *Talking Writing*: "Unleashed" by Jane McCafferty; "Night Fishing" by Sara Hubbs; "Storms of the Circus World" by Lorri McDole; "Paige" by Drew Ciccolo; "Confined to Quarters" by Marianne Goldsmith; "Camera Obscura" by Rebecca Schumejda; "Sacred Touch" by Julie Evans; "Dispatches from the Land of Well" by Jamie Passaro; and "Why Going Crazy Isn't Just a Good Story" by Martha Nichols.

For information about this title or to order other books and/or electronic media, contact the publisher:

Talking Writing, Inc.
P.O. Box 381277
Cambridge, MA 02238
talkingwriting.com
twbooks@talkingwriting.com

Library of Congress Control Number: 2018914982

ISBN: 978-1-7329748-0-7

Printed in the United States of America

Cover and Interior design: 1106 Design

Publisher's Cataloging-In-Publication Data
(Prepared by The Donohue Group, Inc.)

Names: Nichols, Martha, 1958- editor. | Vonnegut, Mark, writer of supplementary
    textual content.
Title: Into sanity : essays about mental health, mental illness, and living in between :
    a Talking Writing anthology / edited by Martha Nichols ; preface by Mark
    Vonnegut.
Description: Cambridge, Massachusetts : Talking Writing Books, [2019] | Some
    essays previously published in Talking Writing magazine. | Includes bibli-
    ographical references.
Identifiers: ISBN 9781732974807 | ISBN 9781732974814 (ebook)
Subjects: LCSH: Mental illness. | Mentally ill—Family relationships. | Mental
    health. | LCGFT: Essays.
Classification: LCC RC454 .I58 2019 (print) | LCC RC454 (ebook) | DDC
    616.89—dc23

To all with open hearts and minds

TABLE OF CONTENTS

INTRODUCTION

～

LIVING IN BETWEEN

MARTHA NICHOLS

How do I write about mental illness?

That's the question raised by *Into Sanity*, a collection of remarkable essays. It's been close to three years since I read the original drafts by contributors, and yet, as their editor and fellow writer, I remain awed by the honesty here. Grappling with the meaning of internal confusion requires sharp self-examination as well as vulnerability. It takes courage. It's like shadowboxing a crowd of thousands.

Some contributors vividly describe sudden descents into the shadows. Others detail what it means to be a family member or witness to someone else's turmoil—or the legacy of illness that ripples down the generations. The essays move far beyond treatment advice, self-help glosses, and clinical labels. Instead, they convey the lived reality of being mentally ill and the long slog back to personal stability.

While there have been scores of memoirs about mental illness or its treatment, *Into Sanity* contains a multitude. That's what makes this anthology so unusual and important—many voices, many experiences, no single story. Memoirs by individual authors tend to emphasize the recovery arc. They're narratives in which the sick, after enduring trials and tribulations, get well. But the contributors of *Into Sanity* come at mental illness and wellness from a variety of perspectives, capturing what these protean states feel like without always providing triumphant resolution.

If you've experienced mental illness and recovery—and every phase in between—you may recognize yourself in these stories. *Into Sanity* is meant to provide validation for what you've gone through. It's also meant for those who worry about the behavior of a loved one. Suicide attempts. Street drugs. Explosive bouts of rage or obsessive checking. A spouse who won't get out of bed. A child who cuts herself. You may want to help, but end up shoved away or irritated or wrestling with your own realization that there are no quick fixes.

If you work with the mentally ill, *Into Sanity* will be especially valuable. Psychiatrists, psychologists, nurses, social workers, interns, medical students, and other clinical professionals spend hours observing patients and their families from the outside. But the stories here are snapshots from the inside, offering entrée to internal states that are rarely captured by intake interviews.

You'll find intelligence, beauty, compassion, even comic flashes in these pages. You'll find love. People recover, but they still feel fragile, getting necessary support from doctors, ministers, family, and friends. *Into Sanity* delves into the flip sides of mental illness and health, shaking up the received wisdom like bits of glass in a kaleidoscope. These writers offer glimpses of new color and light, revealing much more than the arid language of diagnosis, and I'm proud to be among them.

How do I know if I'm mentally ill?

Well, maybe you don't. I don't know where I exist on the spectrum of delusions and compulsions and extreme sensitivity. I'm living in between, as I suspect most people are if they've brushed up against the illness but consider themselves basically healthy and connected to life.

It's not a matter of *I'll know it when I see it*, as if the signs of mental illness are as obvious as shouting "Fire!" in a crowded theater. Take all the family stories I've heard, the ones that supposedly foreshadow disaster, which may or may not be true. My mother would regale my brother and me with possible suicides among her Sicilian relatives or the vendetta against her in Albany, New York—little of which has ever been confirmed. Meanwhile, she didn't tell us about the time as a teenager she tore her own closet apart. Our uncle told us that, as we sat drinking bad coffee in a café a few years ago near her assisted-living facility. Neither my brother nor I reacted much; we'd long since learned to control ourselves.

The only thing I know for sure is how easy it is to collect these stories and to reconfigure them. I wasn't kidding when I said shadowboxing with a crowd of thousands.

An outsider looking at my family might wonder what the trouble was. On my mother's side at least, they were solidly middle-class. Sure, my great-grandfather Vincenzo Valenti started off a coffin-maker outside Palermo, but his immigrant son James ended up an architect in Albany. My mother, Elizabeth Antonia Valenti ("Betty Ann"), was born in 1935, his second child with his first wife Martha. That Martha had French Huguenot roots in upstate New York going back to the late 1600s.

Martha died young, however, when little Betty Ann was only eight. By my mother's account, this early death traumatized her. The adults wouldn't let her or her younger brother go to the funeral; her quick-tempered Sicilian father berated and belittled her. This was explanation enough for why my mother became "sick" (in the family parlance), for her artistic talent mixed with paranoia and screaming rages. She even named me for her own lost mother, a burden I accepted without question as a child.

But my mother was also grateful when a psychiatrist finally gave her a bipolar diagnosis in the 1970s. I was grateful, too. I still am, a good five years after her death. My mother never denied that she needed help. As a young mom in the early sixties, when we'd moved to California, she saw doctors and dutifully took her prescribed medications. Over the decades, she burned through Valium, Haldol, Lithium, Elavil, Wellbutrin, and Depakote, among others.

She was originally labeled schizophrenic, and her first stay in a psych hospital happened circa 1963—after she mixed Mellaril with red wine, I've been told. This sent her into a seizure on the kitchen floor with five-year-old me looking on, although I have no memory of it. It's another shadow I can't stop boxing.

Like so many children of manic depressives—the old evocative term—I have genetic residue. I've struggled with low-level depression since college, alternating with long spells of what clinicians refer to as "hypomania." On the Valenti side, many others in my family have been hospitalized for depression and its bipolar variations, alcoholism, drug addiction, psychotic breaks. And my father's side includes its own unstable mix. The son of a Norwegian immigrant from South Dakota (his mother) and a part-Creole gambler from New Orleans (his father), my dad used to say one of his Norwegian uncles jumped off a silo—probably a suicide, although the Vold family called it an accident.

I've spent decades rationalizing the ancestral threads of mental illness, as if somebody going haywire is inevitable. I've gained many insights over the years, but ironically, the intellectualizing that happens in therapy doesn't serve my writing. Therapeutic insight takes you only so far; ditto for the most effective meds. Maybe writing is just another defense, but I don't care. The contributors to *Into Sanity* delve into the illness with the intensity of existential detectives, and their personal stories are the only things that reflect my notion of it.

I've abandoned faith in direct causation, although I used to be more scientifically inclined. When I left college with a BA in psychology, I worked for a year as a research associate in the affective disorders clinic at the University of Pittsburgh's Western

Psychiatric Institute. Before then, I'd assumed I would become a clinical psychologist. But that year—spent with patients on suicide watch, laid-off steelworkers, single mothers from the Hill District enduring the first hits of the Reagan era—seared me. I didn't feel so different from them. In fact, I felt myself sliding toward them. Then I began developing the detachment required to function in a place like Western Psych, and I got scared.

In my early twenties, I had yet to reckon with my own history. I figured I could hurdle right over that mess by becoming a professional headshrinker. Then some survival instinct kicked in, and I knew I wanted to be a writer. I couldn't stay there if I wanted to get at the roiling undercurrents in myself.

Nobody would say my father's mother was mentally ill. A physically tough woman well into her eighties, she had a laconic Norwegian accent. When my mom went to the psych ward the first time, my grandmother came out on a Greyhound bus from Denver to take care of us. She was strict, forcing my brother and me to eat canned hash and day-old oatmeal. Looking back, I think she might have been furious. Her weak daughter-in-law had let herself fall apart, abandoning her beloved son and grandkids. I remember little except hating her food.

Still, my grandmother was eccentric. I have to wonder about her girlhood on that grim farm in the Dakotas, the aching winter cold, the burning sun and loneliness. She ran away in her teens, was a ranch cook in Wyoming, married and quickly divorced two ne'er-do-wells. She ended up in a Denver apartment with my father, a single mother who worked full-time in a laundry.

When I was older, she told me she missed the wide-open skies of the Plains. She complained about the Rockies "blocking the sky," as if it were herself being blocked. She refused to see doctors or to wear glasses, reading the newspaper through a big magnifying glass.

She must have had her own undercurrents. She always seemed to be arguing with something, as I do to this day. I sensed all that bright light with nowhere to go. Even if the biological basis of mental illness is clear to me, there are real mysteries of personality and circumstance—sparks amid the undercurrents.

Medical professionals of all sorts didn't listen to my mother. I didn't believe her paranoid opinions about anything involving Italians or my relatives, but I never questioned her mood swings or her fear or her chronic pain once she'd undergone a series of failed spinal fusions. Except for a few well-loved social workers and psychiatrists, most doctors and nurses looked down at her, penalizing her for overly melodramatic complaining. They wrote her off as a crazy lady.

When she felt good, though, my mother was one of the most playful and passionate people I've ever known. She was the young mom all my friends wanted to be around. She was a visual artist, a seriously talented one, who poured huge gobs of color and spirit into her creative work. She never had much material success, but my mother would say art saved her life. And it did. I grew up with her passion for spending hours a day on a painting—or, in my case, a story—and that faith in the power of creativity to find meaning in confusion has stuck.

*How do we write about mental illness
and every state of being in between?*

When I began this introduction, I was going to say we need to "attack the problem" of mental illness, but that sounds too angry. It's short-sighted, as if I've tapped a direct channel to the zeitgeist of all those who think mental illness is a character flaw or just a matter of donning a better attitude.

I sound angry anyway. I'll acknowledge that openly now, because I've been angry most of my life. If I didn't have my anger, I'd feel helpless, resentful, blind to the suffering of others, and I'll admit I've felt those things, too. But I also know that anger isn't the only response to handling the social stigma against the mentally ill. Anger is a starting place, as is despair or improbable joy.

Some of us survive just fine. We are the resilient ones, in the language of therapy. Others rattle apart, put themselves back together, then rattle apart again. I think they're resilient, too, but their bravery is often hidden from the rest of the world, revealed only when writers like the contributors to *Into Sanity* tell their stories. Those colored bits of glass shake around, but not always in pretty formations. Sometimes, it's more like staring at a tumble of trash in a dumpster.

My mother never found the one magic pill that fixed everything for good, because life happens as you flail. If your emotions are too big, few people ask why everybody else's are so small. At the same time, we humans are drawn to flashes of brilliance in words and paint, to big-screen grins or fisted hands shaking at an oppressive universe. We love those who seem larger than life, until we pull back, worried, quick to damp down any sparks in ourselves.

Fear and guilt fuel much of the cultural ignorance about mental illness. Bureaucrats and politicians often ignore suffering if it appears to have no real-world cause, and too many people retreat behind *No way—that could never happen to me or anyone I know.* This collection takes the opposite stand. Our intention is to shine a light on what can seem strange or irreparable. *Into Sanity*, a gathering of unique voices, underscores how much mental illness—and wellness—are essential parts of the human condition.

Acknowledgments

I'm deeply pleased to be launching Talking Writing Books with this anthology. *Into Sanity* never would have come together without the support of its contributors, and I couldn't have asked for a better group of writers to work with. The topic is a personal one for me and for them, which can be tricky during the editing process. But these are courageous writers. The effort involved in pinning down what they believe and know was often emotionally taxing—but the reward has blossomed into amazing stories. Thank you all. Again.

The anthology project began with a 2016 personal essay contest at *Talking Writing*, the digital magazine and Boston-area nonprofit organization I cofounded in 2010. The topic was mental illness, and Mark Vonnegut agreed to be our guest judge. He has written two memoirs about his own mental illness—*The Eden Express* (1975) and *Just Like Someone Without Mental Illness Only More So* (2010)—and Mark's unsentimental views and connection to his father Kurt brought in an unusual batch of submissions. "It was truly a privilege to read these entries," Mark told us.

At *Talking Writing*, we decided to collect the best of the submissions, including essays by contest winner Jane McCafferty and finalist Lorri McDole, into our first print anthology. *Into Sanity* is the result. Its 22 contributors come from all over the United States—from California to the Pacific Northwest to the Midwest to the South to New England. Many of them are women and mothers. In addition to this introduction, there's my epilogue: "Why Going Crazy Isn't Just a Good Story," from an earlier *Talking Writing* review of Mark Vonnegut's memoirs.

An independent nonprofit magazine with a small budget has to rely on the dedication of its editors, many of whom donate their time pro bono. Contributing editor Lorraine Berry was my fellow reader of submissions for the 2016 essay contest and an early supporter of the anthology. Managing editor Jennifer Jean administered entries during the contest, and copy editor Erin Goodman turned her sharp eye on the final versions. As always, I thank Karen Ohlson, my editor supreme, for keeping me focused. Another big nod goes to Elizabeth Langosy, TW's cofounder, who championed work about mental illness in the magazine's early years. More gratitude goes to the staff of 1106 Design, especially Michele DeFilippo, Ronda Rawlins, and Brian Smith, for turning this collection of manuscript pages into a book.

And special thanks go to Mark Vonnegut. He was generous enough to write the preface that follows, and I can only emphasize how much he's inspired many of us. In my *Talking Writing* interview with him in 2014, he noted, "Is life random? The details are random." When I asked how you get to truthful writing amid the randomness, Mark said softly, "You watch the details."

Then you let them add up.

Source

"Mark Vonnegut: Too Easy, Dad," interview by Martha Nichols, *Talking Writing*, Spring 2014.

PREFACE

⟢

TELLING THE TRUTH
TO SAVE YOUR OWN LIFE

MARK VONNEGUT

Writing is an all-consuming activity. Mental illness is an overwhelming experience. It's hard to imagine the two not going together. The desire to write and the desire to get well are one and the same. Not everyone can write or write well. The other arts can work as well. Mental illness is being stuck, whether in depression, anxiety, delusion, psychosis, or thoughts of self-harm—yet almost everyone has islands of being well and a desire to be better, to talk to other people. Art, especially writing, is a way to get unstuck, to relate to others, to expand the moments and islands of being well.

Not everyone wants to get well. I've had magic powers that at times were not entirely unenjoyable. But among the other things meds do when they're working is to make art and the human contract more accessible. We're social animals, like it or not. Choosing to have as little as possible to do with other people is a reasonable choice as long as it is a choice. My hunch is that someone making such a choice would have a strong wish to write about it.

Writing about mental illness is almost invariably powerful because the experience is so powerful and the victories—large and small—are so hard fought. The battles bring out strengths and weaknesses writers may not have known they had. Writing has a revelatory purpose and a therapeutic effect. It raises writers up and out of the muck. They're rightfully proud, and we are rightfully made larger, more empathetic, and a little braver.

All great art, especially writing, comes from people at risk who are telling the truth to save their own lives. That truth is what we and they feel and resonate with. This is particularly evident in the stories that follow. The most common words and themes throughout are about being alone and loneliness. Behind every story is a hope of being read and less alone. Even if such stories are partly or nearly entirely dark, we learn a lot. Our world and empathy grow.

Having written a story or a poem, whether or not it's good, is an enormously positive act—an island of wellness that can be expanded and lead to other islands. My recovery started in making Christmas tree ornaments and singing along to Sam Cooke's "Bring It on Home to Me." With these stories now published in a collection, they are bigger islands leading up and away from loneliness.

Milton, Massachusetts

November 2018

SNAPSHOTS

I imagined her rushing around those rooms with her cameras, trying to capture it all. The quotidian, miraculous stuff of life. Seeing the gap between what I imagined she'd seen and what she'd been able to capture was heartbreaking.

—Jane McCafferty

UNLEASHED

~~~~~

JANE McCAFFERTY

When I talk to someone "crazy" out there on the street—someone unwashed in a big coat who's been unleashed from their own sanity—I'll sometimes see my mother's face flashing behind them like a light. Before I know it, I'm imagining a history for the person. It's a kind of practice I've developed on behalf of my mother as a way to remind myself not to dismiss people. I might see them as a child, seated at a school desk, raising their hand. Or I try to see them as a newborn.

How surprised they must have been, how betrayed they must have felt, when their illness, whatever it was, drew a curtain over one world and opened up another. I imagine their exhausted loved ones, far-flung, scarred, sorry, just trying to go forward. And then I usually try to talk to the person, making eye contact. I've learned that sometimes you can see through to what's essential in a human being, even when their mind's gone haywire. Look a person in the eye, and unless they've been entirely shattered, you'll often get a glimpse of a soul who's watching, who knows the self on display in the big coat is just one self among many.

⟾

The last time I visited my mother in a psychiatric hospital, she had that look in her eye for more than a few moments. It was almost a conspiratorial wink, though I didn't want in on the conspiracy. It said she understood, if only for a moment, that the whole story about her having just given birth at 78 to Irish triplets who were being cared for by nurses on the fifth floor wasn't really true—even as, in her mania, she believed it and planned a most ornate christening with the triplets in pink-lace gowns, a five-feet-high cake, her favorite priest performing the baptism, and everyone, of course, invited—the nature of her mania being always to include as many as possible, including people she barely knew. She might come up with the name of someone she sat beside at a basketball game fifteen years ago and insist we find him and extend the invitation.

Miss Evelyn, the African American woman from Baltimore who was her roommate, sat nodding, like a member of a congregation listening to a beloved preacher. *Mmmm hmmm. Got that right. Mmmm hmmm.* Miss Evelyn was in her sixties, with silver glasses and a kind, inquisitive face. It was difficult to see what her illness was—probably she'd been drugged into submission, but the two of them were a team, living for weeks together in that unkempt hospital room, having horrible hospital meals (small clumps of mush and meatloaf, all of which they were vocal about appreciating) at a tiny table, sharing utensils, eating food off each other's plates (an image that would have horrified my hyper-hygienic mother when in her "right mind"), their bare knees touching underneath like blank faces. As they talked, their eyes locked. Theirs was a brand of wild intimacy. I envied it. It highlighted for me my own separateness, my careful friendships, the distance I maintained with other humans. What friend would I sit with this way, knees touching, eyes searching?

I was stationed in a different world, observing them. They loved spending time together and had each other's backs, as Miss Evelyn said. There was a good feeling in that room, though if you judged it through a conventional lens, you wouldn't notice. But it knocked me into a state of wonder. It wasn't hard to see my mother on what amounted to an island I could only visit as a mystified tourist. I'd probably been a mystified tourist since my infancy, when my mother, having given birth to me, crashed into a devastating depression; I had to be handed to others so she could go to the hospital for months.

A few years ago, my friend's husband, a psychologist, said that they've quantified how depression in the face of a mother regarding her infant is in essence a kind of imprinting. The infant wants, above all, to be born into communion. In the face of a severely depressed mother, the infant discovers the face as a wall, as rejection, and turns inward. Being with my mother when she wasn't well was an old, familiar experience for me—lit by the feeling that she was ultimately unknowable, unreachable, and someone from whom I needed protection.

Part of me was always glad my mother found a way to cast off the shackles of her ordinary consciousness. My mother's manic episodes began in her late teens in the early 1950s. This was the beginning of a long walk in and out of radical peaks and valleys, both of which would require hospitalizations.

In some of her episodes, she believed she was pregnant with Jesus.

I remember getting the call with this news when she was nearing sixty. "There's been a miracle," she whispered. In a slightly louder voice I recognized as already altered: "I'm pregnant."

"You *can't* be pregnant." A light shot through me like the headlight of a train I knew I couldn't stop.

"But I am! I'm pregnant with You Know Who."

Unfortunately, I did know who.

"How could that possibly be true?" I said, chills running across my shoulders, my body on high alert, the landscape of my sunlit bedroom shifting, and my face growing hot.

She was calling me from an outdoor shower. She had to make the call there so my father, who was in the cottage, wouldn't hear. "You know he's a worrier." (A terrific understatement.) He wasn't ready to hear the news, she said, but he would be when she was "further along." It was a miracle like the one that happened to Mary.

I paced in my room, with a mixture of fear and excitement, as if some of her mania was being transferred to me. At the same time, I felt fiercely protective of her, as I have all my life, and so felt strong and ready to battle enemies she was sure to inspire. The cold eyes of strangers. Or the nurse from the state hospital on the phone one night who described my mother as "dancing like a crazy motherfucker"—even after they'd shot her full of Thorazine—because she was wildly walking up and down the hall, shouting at people. While I understand the nurse might have been new or burned-out, hearing this hurt like a punch to the gut. I thought of all she didn't know about my mother, who was not some crazy motherfucker, but my mother.

~~

I sat down on my bed, leaning back on a pillow, listening. "Maybe you forgot to take your meds, Mom?"

"Jesus Christ, how can you say something so stupid, you know I never forget to take my goddamn meds!"

She was ushering in the Christ child, but this didn't mean she couldn't cuss. And it was true: Sometimes, the meds weren't strong enough and needed to be adjusted. But she was not "non-compliant." She felt grateful for her Lithium, for the way it allowed her to live a so-called normal life most of the time. Without Lithium and devotion from family, most especially my father, she would have ended up homeless.

~~

Those conversations about the coming birth of Jesus were strangely easy for me to enter, in part because I felt, when she was rising into a manic state, she was more *herself.* Or rather that she was allowed to access a part of herself that heavy medication stamped out. True, medication saved her life and allowed her to be, on the surface, a conventional mother in a suburb who packed great school lunches, worked part-time jobs through the years as a teacher or librarian, in a bridal shop, once behind the counter in a breakfast place—an often brilliantly funny woman who we called "the human jukebox" because she knew the lyrics to hundreds of songs by heart. Before she married, she'd worked for Catholic Charities and volunteered as a teacher in a women's prison.

Her great charm came shining through when she was in public. She was adored out there for her warmth and high spirits.

But she carried a deep frustration under her skin that often became anger, and I always wondered if the source of this was partly the straitjacket of all that medication. The price she had to pay for being normal. When she went into the hospital during my childhood, we were told she "needed a rest." But even at five years old, I sensed there was more to it than that, and for years my prized possession was the leather turtle purse she sewed me in Arts and Crafts at the state hospital. I wore it around my neck as if it contained the heart of a story nobody would tell me. Every night, I got down on my knees, my mother beside me, and prayed for three doctors: Doctor Melker, Doctor Boudre, and Doctor Anstriecher. All three psychiatrists my mother adored and depended on, though I didn't know that at the time. I can't even recall if I thought it was odd to pray for three doctors every night.

And really, what could a small child be told that made any sense?

One of my earliest memories is riding in the backseat of a car with her at the wheel, crying with joy—telling me how happy she was, how beautiful life was. I was three or four years old. She wanted me to see her and kept turning from the road, asking me if I was happy, too. I don't remember what I said. I remember feeling alone. The atmosphere of the car was charged with something I couldn't name. I don't know if I felt I was in danger. I don't know if my memory of holding on to the ledge of the door is invented. I do remember looking ahead, through the front windshield, out at the road, trying to see what it was she saw.

⁓

When I was older, a young adult, and her Lithium stopped working, when she was rising toward that familiar state of ecstatic joy, her voice became, to my ears, more real, more embodied. A rich, expansive undertone entered her speech. I felt her telling me the story of her miraculous pregnancy was the only way she could translate a mysterious ecstasy that allowed her to feel a deep love for everyone, for existence itself. There is a stage in mania that seems identical to a mystic's understanding of everything being ultimately connected, of intense and inexplicable joy being at the very foundation of what is. I've seen that in her face many times.

But where a mystic rises toward divine union, a truly manic person usually rises toward danger. She'd get on the phone and ask people, "What do you need? What do you want most of all that you can't have? Because I'm going to get it for you. A car? New furniture? A trip around the world? You deserve it!" (My father learned quickly to hide the credit cards.) She'd call lawyers and a judge she was friends with in order to sue a man who'd sold her a bad pair of shoes forty years ago. If she got in a car, she'd drive it as fast as she could.

When you tried to tell her no, you can't drive or leave the house, and no, you're not carrying triplets, twins, or Jesus, calling her out like that brought on rage. When she got to that state, she had to be committed, because, as we had seen too many times, she'd get higher and higher, wilder, full of oddly brilliant (and sometimes very funny) rapid-fire speech and strength, and then, if she weren't brought down slowly with chemical cocktails, crash-land into paralyzing darkness. Obliterating depression.

Once, a few years ago, I found about forty photographs she'd taken with throwaway cameras. They were all of the most ordinary things in the ordinary house. A chair, the floor, a couch, the door, a blanket, a lamp. She had taken them in a recent manic state. She had looked one day at a chair she'd lived with for thirty-odd years, suddenly apprehending its illumined essence, its impossible beauty, something that had been waiting for years to be seen.

I imagined her rushing around those rooms with her cameras, trying to capture it all. The quotidian, miraculous stuff of life. Seeing the gap between what I imagined she'd seen and what she'd been able to capture was heartbreaking. The loneliness of those fiery perceptions—of anyone's perceptions, really. These impossible translations we're all trying to make, each one of us on a spectrum of mental health and illness, most of us haunted by all we'll never find a way to communicate—even to ourselves.

The pictures also reminded me of how asleep we often are to our landscapes, to the present as it breathes in the days of our lives. How mania—at least her kind of mania, before it was full-blown and required police to usher her into the back of a cop car so as to escort her into a hospital—resembles enlightenment. Who wouldn't want to wake in the morning and feel their heart break for the beauty of the wooden desk chair by the window? Writing that, I feel the mystery conjured by the words; the image gathers light. *Wooden desk chair by the window in the morning.* The thing itself. What good poetry can deliver. But too often, I'm dulled to familiar trees, faces, my very own breath. There's a price to pay for the kind of culturally induced sanity that is a prerequisite for efficiency, the mind that keeps the wheel turning.

I used to wish we could bottle whatever it was she felt when she was manic but not yet dangerous. And now, at eighty, it seems this is where she's landed. After her kidneys began to fail six years ago, she had to go off Lithium. My brother figured out some new medications for her. She's in the state that resembles a mystic much of the time now—a mystic with dementia coming to obliterate her, slowly, in stages. She sings everyone's praises, names every particular good thing that happens, despite her utter dependence on others for eating, bathing, using the bathroom. She is grateful for that beautiful bowl of rice pudding her neighbor brought her. She weeps with love at the mention of my father or any of her old friends, especially the dead ones. But she doesn't follow those emotions into a story of loss. She comes right back to the present. Praises a cloud sliding by the window. If I ask her what she wants for dinner, it's like I'm asking her what she wants to do in ten years. She's wedded to the moments as they come.

So, who is she? Who are we, if tinkering with brain chemistry can change us so radically? Are we anybody? Are we a potential crowd? Right now, I can see my mother's familiar soul shining in her face, despite the devastation to mind and body, so I'd argue yes, we're souls, we're carrying our souls forward. We're mysteries.

Some people will luck into a genetic pool where ordinary consciousness is never threatened. Their selves will seem stable entities, unless they look harder and come to understand that nobody and nothing is "stable," that we are all at the mercy of a universe where everything changes. Some people will be better at believing in their constructed identities. Loyal to the story of who they are, chemistries balanced, their identities will seem more coherent. I envy that substantial crowd, but really, is there any such thing as a coherent human being, when you really look hard? I think on some level we all know there isn't, which is part of why we feel so uncomfortable about those whose incoherency is so flagrantly on display.

I had a lot of mothers. The blue-eyed beauty who sang and inspired lifelong friendships and devotion from family. The one on the couch, laid low, telling me she couldn't wait to die. The storytelling comedian. The one with the temper I feared. The one who tried to usher Jesus in again. The one who made us excellent meals, made sure we had clothes, drove my brother to hockey practice, picked me up from school even when her back was bad. And now the eighty-year-old with Parkinson's dementia who needs 24-7 care. Her short-term memory's been blasted, and now, some pieces of long-term memory are starting to fade. Another self will be ushered in soon enough.

I wish my mother had not suffered so terribly from this illness. I wish I'd never been that child hearing her say she'd rather have a limb sawed off than endure another serious depression. This was much too high a cost for those states of joy where she seemed, strangely, most herself. But when I'm saying I wish she had no mental illness, it's almost like saying I wish she'd been a different person, which is almost like saying I wish I didn't exist. Which has sometimes, but not often, been true.

TRY ENDING THIS WAY

BETH RICHARDS

You can try ending this way. The pills are shiny and black, and they nestle in your palm like oblong beads, like finely formed beetles. One at a time, they produce a soft down pillow inside the head, just behind the eyes—while you sleep, they carefully, like a sculptor working softwood, shave away the tendons that span memory and pain. The pain eases, the memory vanishes, at least for a while. You vanish.

Two at a time, and the mind's soft pillow turns to honey butter, slippery and sticky and a little too sweet. Three bring murky, dry-mouthed forgetting. Six take you on the circus walk, the tightrope between breathing and ceasing, a teetering between the two worlds. Seven, eight, nine, and you'll fall off the rope, into the welcome, dreamless, memory-less abyss.

You do not feel the lump in the throat that some predict, the sudden hesitation, the butterfly-stomach moment of stepping off the wire, heading downward, the wire whipping upward, suddenly unburdened. You know most people's mistake is taking too many, puking them up. So you calculate the best you can, convert your body weight from pounds to kilograms, the measure of your life. Even so, you heave yourself awake, the black gelatinous mass smeared across the sheets. You have saved yourself by accident, by your lifelong inability to sleep on your back. Your arms are too heavy to push you up from the bed, out of your own muck. When you are more awake, you will remove this messy evidence.

⟜

You can try ending this way. Starvation is quiet and neat—not so bad, you tell yourself. The first days bring the ravenous, obsessive hunger, the belly's gnawing at itself, the burning in the throat. But the hunger, at least for food, subsides. After a while, there is only dull fatigue, a companionable ache behind the eyes. You worry that people will notice, but they don't. A few even compliment you on "looking good." It helps that you don't make a fuss. It helps that people see only what they wish to see. Your shoulder blades stick out like angel wings, stark beauty sculpted from your slender, waning days. Anytime now, a strong breeze will take you up, up, away from here.

But they are stubborn, these cells of yours. Underneath your skin lie tenacious muscle, viscera, and bone, a lifetime supply. You may not want to stick around, but they do, and they wrap a miserly mitt around every caloric offering, the comic dabs of food you eat. You dream of swimming in ice-cream sundaes. You see patty-pan squash in the laundry basket, pork chops like greasy filigree on streetlights. When you still don't eat, your cells change course. They give up trying to seduce you with hot-fudge dreams, the scent of fresh fruit in the shower, and resort to force. They push you to the ground, beam garish colors from the wrong objects: yellow tap water, pink grass, faces the jade green of Palmolive liquid soap.

Someone fingers your fleshless bones, says, "You are not okay." Before you can shape your mouth around a rebuttal, an IV sends sugar directly into your blood. Your cells hip-slip a victory dance, as your animal self roars up and demands to be fed. Honey dissolved in warm herbal tea ricochets around your mouth, fires point-blank into your brain. Food makes its way into you: a bite of butter-touched egg; a ring of tender pasta; a curl of briny, pink shrimp. Though your pain is the same sharp insistence it always was, your angel wings retract. Politely say "Thank you." Chew and swallow. For dessert, look for something more effective.

⌒⌐

You can try ending this way. The blades you use at work to cut little jigsaws of words into the galleys, they are just right. When no one is looking, you wrap a sharp new one in tissue and put it in your shirt pocket. Its shape comforts as you take the print off the linotype, wax, and then position the corrections neatly with the tip of the X-Acto knife. You admire its pointed precision, anticipate the ease with which it will sink into your skin.

Because your endings thus far have not gone as planned, you decide to do some research. This is before the Internet, and so you must be content with the neighborhood library, the deepest recesses of the stacks. Veins carry blood back to the heart, arteries carry blood away. You choose arteries. But arteries are more muscular than veins, and veins are closer to the surface. You choose veins. *Gray's Anatomy* shows the arm's vascular schemata: basilic and cephalic and antebrachial. You contemplate the different strata—corneum, lucidum, granulosum. You whisper the names as you finger the wrapped blade, though it is not quite clear to you which layer you are supposed to cut through or beyond. You watch a couple of teen angst movies, deduce that the best approach is lengthwise, not across. You must open enough surface so that your blood's pesky platelets don't accumulate and gum up the show.

You think that cutting through the layers of papery skin on the inside of your arm will be swift, just like the blade slices through the magazine galleys. But your skin turns out to be tough stuff. It resists, it stretches, it pulls miserably this way and that before succumbing. There is the welling up of blood—globulus and sapphire red; you expect that. What you don't expect is the sear of pain that runs up your arm and into the very center of your brain, a sensation so weighted that your head snaps back. You drop the blade, stunned—you, who were too numb the week before to feel your fist going through the sheetrock wall.

You try again, steadying yourself against the pain this time. It still hurts, but you breathe through it. You think of pushing bodies away from yours. You think of women in labor. The knife slices through—pay dirt—and you suddenly have what seems to be a lapful of blood. It is warm and curiously both thin and thick. It stinks. It also clots swiftly, decisively. And you understand that even your considerable tolerance for pain won't get you to this ending.

Your body's endorphins flare in full force. A calm as warm and sweet as a nip of neat whiskey washes over you. You place your palm on the wound. The tension that prods you like an electric current has disconnected. You breathe again, deeply. You experiment. The body is exquisitely tuned, and you discover that barely piercing the skin with the sharp blade brings the flooding response, the swelling up of blood, the release of your own inner drugs, always available and always free.

The first cuts take a while to heal, and you worry that the bandage will alert someone. You make up a plausible story—a careless movement with a gardening tool—and it fools everyone except one friend, who stares you down, says, "I don't think so." You try to avoid her, but she calls, then stops by your house, hands you the business card of a counselor. You assure her you're fine. You watch her leave, then blot with the card's sharp corner, watch how the blood tracks the pattern of fibers in the stiff paper. Although the weather is supremely hot and humid that summer, you are always cold. Anemic? You wonder. With obsessive precision, you vary the ways you try to manage the pain: beer on Saturday, church on Sunday. Sprinting until you can't stand up on Monday, Wednesday, Friday. Small divots of the blade on Tuesday—just enough to make the endorphins come, to ensure the release.

Thursdays, late afternoon, you begin to set aside time to talk with the woman whose card your friend gave you, the brown-spotted card you dig out of the trash one night when you look at yourself, your marked skin, in the mirror.

⟍

You can try letting someone else end you. She's tall and good-looking, in a handsome sort of way, a sheaf of dark-brown hair angled at the chin. You are fascinated by every inch of her but especially her ankles, which have not one but two delicate bones, the top one a tiny calcium triangle. She began her mysterious embryonic life as a twin, she says, but was born a singleton. You wonder what other person remains absorbed within her, whether it drives the contradictory moods that both lure and repel you.

You drink a lot, and when you drink, you do anything she says, which, this night, is to go out to a club. She wants to slow dance, even though you don't dance. She loads the jukebox with sweet, forlorn, deep-bellied songs, Patsy Cline and Hank Williams. You can't recall the songs' names, but you can still feel their twinge, the string they thread and then draw tight between you and her. You forget how much you are drinking, and you don't care, because even though you are almost too drunk to dance, you can feel her in your arms, supple and sinuous and warm and—for once—her "no-no" and "yes-yes" cancel out.

You think that you are meant for each other, even though she doesn't see that; you believe the dancing proves it. Except that as you're drinking—which leads to finding more slow songs on the jukebox, which leads to the slow sweet swaying in the center of the floor, all by yourselves—you manage to notice where you are. A country-western bar, and not one that caters to girls dancing with each other, to Hank Williams or anyone else. You realize that the two of you are dancing all alone with each other because everyone else is staring, and that the stares are getting harder and hotter, like bubbles simmering in a saucepan just before they rise to a boil.

She says, "We'd better go." And almost before you feel the pressure of her long fingers on the small of your back, you are hurtling through the door, across the parking lot, toward her small convertible that looks very far away. The footfalls you hear behind you aren't friendly and not nearly as drunk as you'd like them to be. They come closer, the rhythm of the steps a tense counterpoint to the pounding of your heart in your ears, the ragged snaps of your breath.

Her long legs reach the car before your shorter ones do, and she slams the car into gear before her door is completely closed or you are fully inside. You hold on. She puts the pedal to the floor. The car roars up, peels past the bearded, burly men caught a bit off guard by your surprising speed, by her mechanical aplomb.

Later, she says they probably weren't serious when they said they'd be happy to teach you *bitch perverts* a lesson. She concedes, as you glare over cold Waffle House hash browns that you stir and don't eat, that it was "a bit of a close call." She gives you her best smile—all dimples and promise—says that she knew you could run fast, but baby, you were like a jackrabbit, zaggin' and a-ziggin'. You don't ask if she heard what the massive beard-face said into the air behind you as you ran. *Beat the shit out of you. Spread those legs. Make you a real woman.*

You thought you'd do anything for the chance to merge your skinny, singular bones with hers. But you won't tell her this, won't tell her the terror that tore through you. Won't tell her that someone had already made a real woman out of you, and how you could not live through that again. Not for her, not for anyone. You study her, hands moving like a flurry of birds, warm double-ankle sweeping under the table to find yours, eyes alight with the evening's adventures.

She's eaten all her food, while it was still hot. And you wonder if the twin within her, cheated out of a real life, speaks from within her bones, calls to her to do these things. She is smart, quotes Shakespeare and Rilke and Sexton. She wrote a poem, comparing you to a seashell that chewed itself from the inside out. You adore that she wrote a poem about you. You hate its truth. She leans across the Formica table, extends a long finger, taps your cheek. You feel every cell you own shift toward her, this mesmerizing woman who seems to enjoy danger a lot more than she cares about you. You push your congealed plate to the side, push yourself up and away from the table. From now on, you will dance with someone else, elsewhere. Or not at all.

⟜

You can try ending without even trying. There is a canoe, swift-flowing brown river water. In the back of the canoe is the woman you've been dating, not exactly satisfactorily, but it's better than sleeping alone and eating leftover take-out in front of the TV. The first small rapid is larger and more turbulent than you expect, but you're confident. She says she'll rudder the canoe from the back, and so you lean forward into warm sun and cool spray, into thoughts of the end of the day: a spent campfire, her leg damp and warm across you as you gaze at the Milky Way.

But she's been less than truthful about her rudder expertise—as you'll soon find she has been less than truthful about a number of other key details. You hit the second rapid, and the canoe begins to skid, lumbering and unwieldy. She is supposed to pull back on her oar, keep the nose pointed forward, but she panics and digs in instead. You brace hard onto your paddle; the canoe dips and shudders through the rapid, barely upright. You look back at her and realize you want the fuck out of this canoe now, because as much as you've sought death, you don't want it like this: pulverized on a rock and recovered weeks later at the downstream dam, fish-white and nibbled on like Swiss cheese.

The canoe hits the third rapid before you can finish your thought about how you're going to dump this woman out of the canoe, not to mention your life, as soon as you are on dry land. The current carves the river's face and pushes you through a narrowing of raised bank and fern-covered rock. She's not even paddling now; she's frozen. The canoe bangs, wobbles, bucks, and tosses you onto the sliding edge of a sandbar before swirling back around and coming to rest on your lap. Turned sideways, the canoe immediately fills with water and grinds your hips and legs into the sand. Out of the corner of your eye, you see her surface and dog paddle onto the bar, watch her stunned recognition that you're trapped, that as the canoe fills, it's sinking into the sand and pulling you underwater. She digs her hands into your armpits, tries to hold you up as you strain, as you take careful sips of breath by tipping your nose up to the surface like a turtle.

You think, well, shit, you could have saved yourself the trouble of all that other pill-starvation-blade misery and just hooked up instead with this goddamned lying woman with her pathetic paddle skills and lame emergency response. She's screaming and trying to lift the water-filled canoe, which serves only to drive the hull deeper into your hip. You gulp water. You hope that what you've heard about drowning is true: that it's painless after the first underwater inhalation, that as you drift to the other dimension, you'll see glorious colors and unearthly creatures with carved, glinting wings.

And then you pop to the surface and face-plant, right back into the water. Hands grab your shirt collar and waistband, pull—your legs are all weight and no feeling—deposit you on the riverbank, pound your back. You cough up muddy water, chunks of breakfast, about a gallon of rage. Pulling you up out of the water isn't easy; you can hear whoever it is breathing fast and deep. It's not the inept, lying woman doing this, because you see her already on the bank, watching you, her hands small, tight circles in front of her mouth.

Before you imagine pushing the woman away from you in the tent that night, and before you anticipate slamming the car door and walking away forever when you finally get to safe, dry home, you breathe. The air is scratchy with pollen, redolent with the damp of fiddlehead and loam. You roll away from your coughed-up mess, ease your aching, quivering self onto a slight patch of ground warmed by sun that has fought its way through the thick canopy of hickory and sycamore, dogwood and sweet gum. You hear the drone of bees nearby; you can't see the flowers, but a slight breeze lifts their scent to you, warm honey. After the water's turbulence, you're surprised that the sky is so calm and clear, robin's-egg blue, a few puffs of cloud suspended quiet and still.

"I was on the lower trail," says the guy who pulled you from the water. Muscles cable on his thin neck, ripple up and down his legs as he sloshes back out into the current, somehow rights and coaxes the canoe to shore and shoves it into the brush, out of the water's reach. "Heard you yell." You don't remember yelling.

Your empty stomach growls. The sensation returns, pins and blades and needles, to your legs. A patch of blood on your hip seeps watery red-pink through your pants. You are suddenly, overwhelmingly sleepy. But you fight it, fight the sleeping and leaving, the forgetting. You've come so close to what you wanted for so long, only to discover it's not what you want at all.

HURRICANE WARNINGS

MARTHA NICHOLS

My mother had a terrible memory. Sometimes, I thought her misremembering was an aggressive act, the way she'd misinterpret family stories. In 2013, her last year, when we were told she had Alzheimer's, the diagnosis felt sadly anticlimactic. Other disasters had already done their damage: a broken spine that made her wheelchair-bound, arthritis that cramped her artist's hands, mental illness.

One of the last memories I asked her about, at least five years before her death, was the way she used to hit me and my brother with a hair brush when we were little. Her first response was a shrug. *I had to, because one time you kids wouldn't go to sleep. I put you down for a nap, but you just kept getting up. You were so active.*

As I recall, my elderly parents both laughed when she said this.

I was driving. We were in a rental car (too small, my father said) during one of my regular visits to the Bay Area. I'd taken them out to dinner—to Max's Diner, a favorite of theirs, at the

27

top of Crow Canyon Road—and now we were heading home. My parents loved the ride as much as the food. We wound through the northern Californian hills of my childhood, past horse farms and live oaks, far from upstate New York, where my Italian-American mother had grown up.

But when I then asked if they really thought it was okay to hit a child, I saw her misremembering in action. *What! You think that's wrong? Okay, maybe it didn't happen. I don't remember, Martha, please.*

⟶

In September 1960, I don't remember the adults saying *Donna* or *hurricane*. I was two years old, and I wouldn't have known these words. But based on everything I've since read, the adults around me must have been scared. They would have followed the news reports about Hurricane Donna for days as the "storm of the century" battered its way up the east coast from Florida and the Carolinas.

At the time, we were staying at my aunt and uncle's house in Albany, New York. I don't think my father was there, but my mother and seven-month-old brother must have been with me.

It's the first thing I remember, that storm. The morning after Donna blew through, I stood at Aunt Audrey's front door. The screen was open; the sunlight made me squint. I probably saw downed trees and power lines, maybe a broken TV antenna and swampy lawns. I think I wore footie pajamas. Somebody held me back—my mother? an older cousin?—I don't know who, yet I retain the feeling of wriggling, of wanting to break free, of irritation and thrilling wildness.

The most exciting part turns out to be in dispute, however. For years, I was sure I saw the next-door neighbor's roof blow off. The adults may have pointed it out or talked about other roofs down south. It's possible I saw *The Wizard of Oz* when it was broadcast on CBS in 1959, although I would have been only a year old. With Donna, I was a toddler, unable to fathom an abstraction such as a hurricane being in different places over time—so reality surely mixed with fantasy.

My later research indicates that wind speeds weren't very high by the time Donna reached Albany; the National Weather Service reported gusts of 50 mph at most. My mother didn't remember anything about a roof or the storm. Years ago, before my aunt had passed away, I asked her about it, too. In consultation with my uncle, Aunt Audrey thought a nearby roof might have blown off but wasn't sure if it was next door.

Still, I can't write off this first memory as just hearsay or pure fantasy. Recently, I emailed other family members to ask what they recall. Three of my cousins, the children of my aunt and uncle in Albany, confirmed that a nearby roof had blown off (or part of one) on the house across the street. My cousin Tom hadn't yet been born in 1960, but he and his three siblings "did hear the stories."

The roof of that particular house was flat, Tom says, "which is very unusual in our area primarily because of the snow, so if the wind caught it right, it could take off like a wing and get airborne."

He was told it blew over his house and remembers playing with the debris in the backyard when he was little, using it to build forts.

So, it did happen—or I heard about it happening—even if my cousins admit their own memories are fuzzy. (Tom says he was always told it was a tornado.) It's unlikely I saw the roof blow off, but that's what I remember: a roof spinning, circulating like the storm itself.

It's a strange first memory: a big storm, standing in an open doorway, wanting to escape, almost no sense of any other person present. It feels unfair, as if I never asked to remember it—but *unfair*? Can a memory really be unfair? How odd that sounds, how childlike.

The truth that's emerged is sloppy, yet I'm surprised by the grip it has on me. I can't let it go. It's as if I've just realized, at sixty, that I'm not the boss of memory, no matter how much I want to be.

I could invoke Tolstoy's famous opening by noting that all unhappy families remember things in different ways. But when mental illness is part of the family, retrieving and confirming memories is more like a battle with zombies. The memories die but keep coming back to life in unexpected, misbegotten shapes. It's like casting a fishing line into a pool and reeling up a pile of burning leaves. Or a neighbor's roof.

It's hard to trust anything you've heard. After all the fits and starts in my adult career, that's probably why I ended up a journalist.

My mother wasn't diagnosed with bipolar disorder until the 1970s, but I felt ashamed long before that. That's the unfair part;

I never had any control over her moods or what they did to me. I'll admit now that I wish I'd imagined the whole thing about the roof, because the reality points to what I'd rather forget: the dark weather in my own family.

I suspect my mother was frantic as Donna approached, not because I remember it—the absence of both my parents and brother in my recollection is a telling void—but because as I grew older, I knew what it was like to live with her. She had a shifty spark behind her eyes, as if too much light were trapped behind a cloud; spittle would pool at the corners of her mouth. In September 1960, she was only 25, with a baby and a two-year-old, and a hurricane would've been like pouring oil onto a wildfire. Aunt Audrey was the stable one.

But still, well into adulthood, I saw that neighbor's roof twirling in the clouds like Dorothy's house in a tornado. The giddy gut-feeling of standing in my aunt's doorway, lit up by the returning sun and fear and a great big world of possibilities, sticks this memory to many later memories, to my love of clouds and atmospheric disturbances. Maybe even at the age of two, I saw myself riding that roof into the sky, alone.

Sources

"Hurricane Donna 1960" from "Hurricanes in History" page, Hurricane Research Division, National Oceanic and Atmospheric Administration website.

"Hurricane Donna, September 2–3, 1960: Preliminary Report with the Advisories and Bulletins Issued," U.S. Weather Bureau (Department of Commerce), 1960.

"Storm Data, September 1960," U.S. Weather Bureau, 1960.

Tom Hutson, personal correspondence with author, March 14, 2017.

DESCENT

*He looked at me, held my gaze. When I'd told
the ER doctor the previous afternoon that I felt
like killing myself, I never thought about hell.
What kind of believer was I with no hell factored
into the equation?*

—Kristine Snow Millard

NIGHT FISHING

SARA HUBBS

If there is no sleep, then there is no time, and there is no need for sleep training.

This is not a manifesto about co-sleeping. This is about bed-time rituals that don't amount to anything. This is about a bed that was never slept in, about a bassinet I kept next to my bed with my baby in it. This is about a distance that grew between my body and my bed—a space of broken energy between mother and child.

Late in December 2011, we brought our daughter home from the neonatal intensive care unit, a week after she'd been born unable to breathe on her own and had to be resuscitated. I read and reread the warning label on the bassinet in case I'd missed something. It was her first night home, and I stayed with her alone, as I had many nights before while my husband, an emergency physician, worked the overnight shift.

But something held me down, heaviness and stillness on the chest, her chest, this night and many nights that followed. It was Christmas Eve in New York City, my family had all gone home to Arizona, our friends were out of town, and it felt like the eve of another disaster, another morning after, the night the heat went out.

It was freezing outside. I was already afraid to look in the bassinet. I prepared myself for a frozen little body.

I was always worried that someone was going to take her from me, and that morning I couldn't remember how I fed her. Did I feed her? I must have slept, but I only know about the things I did instead of sleep.

My nights were wet. There were bowls of cereal eaten in the dark at the window. There was post-partum blood between my legs and night sweats that left me cold, because winter blankets hurt my skin. There was milk that leaked from rogue breasts and tears siphoned from a dehydrated body.

Notice the worry about food, as if it would disappear. I planned my life around it. There was also an obsession with breast milk, because I feared I wouldn't be able to feed my daughter, as if I didn't know how. One night at two o'clock in the morning, I found myself on the floor, crying next to spilled milk. When I took the shields from my breasts, the clear plastic tubing swept the three-ounce container to the floor. I hated myself.

I tracked her feedings for over three months in a little green notebook, a mom's log, positioned next to the glider. Those were the days of tracking that turned into nights of devotional watching, where ceilings turn into lines, and the lines all led to the floor.

I advise you, please, to clean every speck of dust and bundle of hair from your floors. This is a preventive measure to safeguard against certain cleaning obsessions. I preferred sweeping to holding my baby.

Lean in and look under your radiator.

Also, avoid singing "Baa, Baa, Black Sheep" to your child. It is a song with a motive. It implants itself in your brain and is programmed to turn on as soon as you rest against a soft surface or close your eyes.

Try not to listen to your breast pump; they have been known to mock new mothers. In the quiet cold of late December, the pump will chant/wheeze, *you suck, you suck, you suck* every time the phalanges extrude your nipples to take the liquid that contains your baby's immunity.

Maybe I'm the only one who heard this, the only one who played the record backward.

⟿

Two-and-a-half years after her birth, we moved home to Tucson. We looked for a house to make into a home in a perfectly fine neighborhood on a well-kept street. As we pulled out of the driveway, our realtor told us about a little girl who went missing on the well-kept street. She was reportedly taken from her family via her bedroom window.

I'll tell you a secret. Four years after her birth, our daughter still sleeps in our room. We share a nightlight. She, too, has a bedroom with a window, which I just couldn't and cannot trust.

Listen, this is not an endorsement of helicopter parenting, nor is it an endorsement of attachment parenting. This isn't a treatise against them, either.

Do you want to know another secret? If you don't have a picture of your baby after your birth, you can post a picture of your placenta on Facebook. I find this refreshing.

There is a colony for people like us, a colony of IVs, large needles in spines, baby CPAPs, and little white pills. Little pills that work better than safe words and breastfeeding support groups.

I went to a moms' meet-up once in New York. There were many reasons to be nervous, mainly because I didn't have my "Brest Friend" feeding-device-pillow-strap-thing. *What if I don't get a good latch? Everyone will know I don't know what I'm doing.* I reached into my bag and touched and retouched the emergency bottle of dry formula I carried with me. I positioned myself near a Boppy (better than nothing) in the corner where I barely touched my baby, where I stared at the carpet and hyperventilated. I drowned in the sounds of other moms, wiping tears from my eyes. The vibrations of the room made my body hurt. It was humming, and I needed, I needed to leave. I felt so bad for my daughter.

I need to ask you, have you ever wanted to be the floor? Not just lie on the floor, but also be the rich brown grain of a good hardwood?

Have you ever been suspicious of Skype? I knew there was something weird about my family, about the way their faces looked out at me from the screen. Their silence I took as blame. They wanted to take her from me, too, and at that point, I wouldn't have put up a fight.

This one is delicate. Have you ever recoiled from your own newborn?

Don't leave me alone, I begged.

These are the things that occurred to me after the birth: I couldn't stand in front of the hospital where I birthed our daughter, and I couldn't even get off at the same subway stop. Invisibility can be protective.

Now, I can't enter a hospital without an intense feeling of being jailed, of disaster mode, of a need to drive or run fast or scream loudly. I need to scrutinize everyone, monitor actions and words.

It's also occurred to me that well-meaning people, the pediatrician, the friends who post parenting articles on Facebook, the family who repeat wives' tales, folk remedies, family birth lore, cannot help us. Mother, we are designed to fall through the cracks, because everyone knows what's wrong with you, because nobody knows what's wrong with you. The birth experience is designed for trauma.

The NICU is not designed for families or breastfeeding.

When I was down on our beautiful hardwood floor, when I was stuffing my face with two egg-and-cheese croissants, listening to my neighbor's baby being sleep trained just beyond my wall—my own sleep prevented by nursery rhymes, by dreams that felt like gasps for air—I told my birth story to anyone who would listen like an itch that needed to be scratched.

I told of all 36 hours of induction, all manner of disparaging comments, coercion, of disempowerment. I told of all the ways I was kept from my baby, of all the artificial obstacles to motherhood, until I hated the sound of my own voice. Until I disconnected from the telling, until it became superstition, as if I would compromise my daughter's future state of aliveness by speaking the words *born dead*.

Now, I can only mouth them.

Did this happen? What happened? Was it as bad as it feels? I knew I was to blame. I lacked confidence. I was scared, and my daughter knew it. That's why she had hiccups inside my belly.

One night before her birth, she came to me in a dream. I could see her face clearly. *Is the door open?* she asked. *Yes*, I tentatively replied.

People said I should have had a C-section. Who wants to push a baby out of her vagina anyway? People told me that at least my baby is okay. My aunt told me four weeks after the birth, "It's time to get over it. She's alive."

As I write this, in 2015, it is four *years* after the birth. Don't think for a minute I'm not thankful she's alive, that I'm ignorant of the fact that there are people who have it worse. It's just that when feelings in my body come from nowhere, these supposedly baseless fears I feel are true, they don't come with a sliding scale for pain.

There is a place where mothers like you and me go. It's a place with a curtain, with a bloody handprint hastily swept across the fibers, a curtain between the labor bed and your child's warming bed. The warming bed turned resuscitation bed. It's a place with spotty warm lights and blue babies that plop out of your body. It's a place with chest compressions and miniature laryngoscopes.

Don't worry, there's no skin-to-skin contact in this story; nor is there a cord that pulses to completion. This is about waiting to see if you'll be a mom, and when you realize you are, the complete difficulty of locating yourself in any of it.

Did you know that becoming a mother could come from somewhere behind you or beneath you or in spite of you? Did you know that neither the self you knew before nor the self that comes after actually exists?

There are just starts and stops.

～

Three years to the day of my daughter's birth, she saw the first picture ever taken of her—her face obscured by a breathing apparatus, IVs in her hands and feet wrapped with tape, steadied by a board. She asked me what happened to her, and I told her how hard I worked to get her out.

On my daughter's third birthday, I still dreamed of the birth, although the dreams weren't as frequent anymore. I still startled and felt a tingling sensation radiating from the center of my body when I heard a car honk. I still placed my hand on her chest every night before I went to bed, kissed her forehead—just in case. I still lay in bed, listening to the sound of her breath until I fell asleep. Maybe all parents do this.

On long car rides when she napped, when her body went limp and her head slumped forward, I reached my hand behind me from the driver's seat and bounced her leg, worrying that her trachea would be compressed and she wouldn't be able to breathe. Sometimes, on the highway going 75 miles an hour, I shouted at her until she woke up or took a long inhale and repositioned her head.

I still left nightlights on around the house when my husband worked his overnight shifts at the hospital. Most months he worked up to seven such shifts. I had my cell phone next to my bed. I thought about the steps needed to make an emergency call in the middle of the night, and I reminded myself before I went to bed: swipe right, emergency call button, bottom left. Most nights, I watched TV as late as I could stand because the sound made everything feel normal.

The summer of her third year, we took a trip to San Diego, to Mission Bay, where my family had escaped August in Arizona since I was little. This year, my sister and I sat on our beach towels away from the shoreline while my husband swam with our daughter in the hotel pool. We sat there for an entire afternoon watching emergency workers, police, fire, helicopters, and boats search for a boy who had fallen into the water from a kayak, unable to swim, wearing no life jacket.

The search and rescue gave way to just a search. We watched the lead police officer, the one with the socks pulled up above his calves, eat two full sandwiches on white bread from the passenger side of his SUV. We watched people being interviewed, people falling to pieces, people still swimming in the water—ignorant or indifferent.

We watched as daylight turned to twilight, then into a scene that resembled a painting of night fishermen—darkness surrounding one little boat and one light source seen from the shore. We hit refresh on our search for "foreign exchange student drowned mission bay."

The passenger-ferry rides between two sister hotels across the bay resumed with the boy's body not yet recovered, and my family wanted to go. Shaking, I declared that I would not set foot on the boat and neither would anyone else. That boy's body was still under there, blue, like the surrounding water. Couldn't they see his shape? Couldn't they feel his stillness—the stillness of his chest? Couldn't they feel the emptiness at their bellies?

He was somebody's baby. At least I could be a witness. A witness for his mother who had no idea I was there. The next year, we returned to the bay, and I put flowers in the water for him—for her.

⁓

Every year since the birth, people ask me when I'm going to have another one. I can tell you that even after the pills for post-partum OCD, there is no way to forget. But forgetting is not the point.

Years after the birth, a friend suggested EMDR to deal with my continuing post-partum PTSD. The acronym EMDR stands for Eye Movement Desensitization and Reprocessing therapy. It's a form of psychotherapy that uses the patient's rapid eye movements to help process powerful memories from traumatic events.

I found a therapist who I'll call Judy (it's not her real name). Before and after each session, she asked me, "What's your disturbance level?"

I held the little black tappers, one in each hand. When I was ready, they alternated, vibrating first in my left hand, then in my right hand. Judy asked me to call to mind the most disturbing image or feeling I associate with my daughter's birth.

I closed my eyes and felt the *buzz, buzz, buzz, buzz,* back and forth between my hands. I saw the round, flaccid body of my daughter when she flopped out of mine. She was slippery and a shade of purple-blue. That was the moment I knew something was wrong, when something told me I'd birthed a dead baby.

Judy stopped the tappers and said, "Okay, take a deep breath."

I told her what I'd seen and felt.

"Okay, go with that."

I closed my eyes again, and she started the tappers. In my mind, the image shifted from my daughter, and I saw my husband, the ER doctor, jump in with the nurse to work on her before the NICU staff arrived. He rubbed her body, using tactile stimulation to get her to breathe. She still wasn't breathing, and he was getting ready to intubate her.

I floated above it all, watching. I could see myself in the hospital bed, alone, with the curtain drawn between my bed and the table where he was resuscitating her. Even though they were behind the curtain, I could see it happening.

Judy stopped the tappers and asked me to take a deep breath. She told me I was doing a good job.

I closed my eyes, and the tappers started again. My attention shifted to the doorway, where I saw my baby as they rolled her to the NICU. The doorway was filled with a white light, an incredible light I could feel in my heart. It felt like it contained everything in the entire world.

My eyes were still closed, and the tappers continued. Tears fell silently from my eyes.

"Okay, deep breath. Go with that."

I held my baby's foot. She was hovering above the table, and *she* wanted to be a part of the white light.

Judy asked if I was okay. I said I wanted to continue.

"Deep breath," she said.

I closed my eyes again. I felt the tappers and saw my deceased grandmother sitting in a chair by the window. I knew she was with us.

She was the grandma who helped raise us, who lived just three blocks away. She lost two children of her own: the first, a five-year-old, run over by a truck, the second electrocuted at the age of 33 working on power lines.

She told me, *I just didn't want you to hurt.*

Deep breath. Go with that.

DOG COLLEGE

GREG CORRELL

Author's Note: *In 1970, I was released from juvenile detention in St. Louis, where I'd been raped and tortured for five days by three older boys. I told my brother, who pretended not to believe me, but no one else, and I received no counseling or support. I tried to walk it off, as it were. In 1973, I started college at University of Missouri-Kansas City, where I fell apart, but kept up my grades. After a notebook was found containing my fantasies of self-mutilation, I spoke with university counselors a few times, including the evaluation interview with the woman I describe here. I refused the interviewer's request to go to a psychiatric hospital, because hurting myself was not the main thing. The main thing was my dog, Obie. In this recreation, I give the boy I was a voice, and tell it my way—including what I should have said.*

I used to be a boy who wouldn't walk the dog. Hard to explain the change—I got up, is all. Didn't *want* to, but now I sort of want to, even though—

I'm a good man now. You won't believe me, after I tell you. But I am.

No, I don't want to talk about that yet. I know who the president is. I came to you, right? Well, you called me in, but I came, so let me talk about my dog. Then I'll talk about . . . that other thing.

I *am* calm. I need to do it this way. Okay?

I was a freshman and lived alone, one of those shotgun places, a one-room-through-another deal. I was a loafer—when I got caught up, I slept, even during the day. Fought it all the time—no, I'm a liar right there, see that? I slept even when I had homework. Fucking lazy, then I'd stay up all night, frantic . . . so tired all the time.

I'll calm down.

Friends? I didn't talk to people. Thought I was creepy.

All right, I'll say one thing about that. Back then—that's what this is, really. Back-then stuff. I was *way* too messed-up to have girl sex—girlfriends—I hated it. What? Geez. Jerking, you know, *off* all the time. I *hated* it—I know there's nothing *wrong*—fantasies? No, not . . . I just decided I didn't like it, my . . . dick. I told myself not to—*not* to—but did it anyway—*not to*—*not to*—I was sick. *Not* to—huh?

Yeah, I can stop. Ha. I can *not* say it—*not*.

I thought everyone could see I was f—how sick it was. *I* was.

Yeah, I still feel that way, obviously. Those notebook pictures—last night I was, but I'm not like that anymore. Normally.

I don't sleep right. Last night I got confused, I don't remember exactly, but I almost—I know, but *almost*, so let's go back to my dog. Okay?

Please. Let me tell it my way. I'm sorry. I'll stay calm. I am. I'm sorry.

Thanks. I'll take sips. You're very kind.

My step-dad is a professor here. He wrote a letter last year so I could live off campus. I'm too mature. I was in jail, he knew, and all, about—

I forget what—

Yeah, after jail. He—yeah, my step-dad—he felt it would be humiliating, staying with regular kids in the dorm. I had to live by myself. And Obadiah, the dog. My dog.

I was incorrigible, a runaway, and the cops picked me up. Hmm? About six weeks. It was nothing.

~

I want to tell the truth. *Please.* This table I had, with a linoleum top? Had this thick nickel-steel edge this high, an inch-and-a-half, like—I guess *this* high—and it folded over the top a little. I was stupid about cleaning—okay, still am—so it had dark gummy stuff under the metal. Spilled sauce, God-knows-what from whoever was before me. I used to pick at it with my thumb when I was supposed to do assignments. Pick it out of one thumbnail with the other one—back and forth, like that, see? To get it out. I'd roll it on the table and then get mad at myself for not doing my work.

I had to, you know, discipline myself. I was upset all the time. Used to scratch grime off my neck and look at that under my nails, too, more and more—I left bleeding scratches, like this, see? All over my neck. I know! No, I'm just showing you—more and more—okay! I *know!*

More and more.

Funny. I don't remember what the shower looked like in that place. I must have taken one. I don't remember. Not at all.

Lonely. Yeah. One time, this girl who had the whole third-floor attic place? She stops me in the hall when I was bringing up my bike, says, "I can hear you, you know. At night. In my place." She looked at me with her mouth tight, like this, eyes sideways, and I felt that freeze feeling, but my face was hot. I had to tell the tops of my legs not to, like, buck up.

I nodded. "Yeah, okay, thanks." Kept my face all neutral. She was like, "You shouldn't let me hear you talk about that." So I smiled normal, like this, and said, "Okay." I was being honest but in a way not, too—

I'm going to ignore your questions. I'm not trying to be mean—I *am* calm. Just—you have to make papers and everything, but can you just be human? I'm saying *please.* Then I'll do it, whatever.

See, I still do it, I black, I mean *blank* things out, even instantly. I really didn't get what she said, but when I went inside, I tried to remember what I talk about at night in front of the mirror, what she heard—crying, all that lonely stuff. And hurting myself. Maybe that, too. I might have said that out loud. Not sure. And repeating myself, how I can't make it stop. Couldn't. I'm always like this.

Was, I mean. I don't know what I would do if I couldn't talk in my bathroom anymore.

Right. *Thank you.*

~

My dog Obie, that's what I *really* need to talk about.

She used to pee in the corner of the kitchen, by the door. I'd get mad, but I didn't hit her. I mean, I swatted her with a rolled-up paper, like you're supposed to, when she pooped inside, which she hardly did because I walked her twice a day, before class and after dinner. Sometimes I took her to class, tied her to the bike rack, and she pooped and peed there.

All I ever did was go to class and work-study. And evening yoga, if I wasn't nervous. To get my breathing right, be normal in class and all.

Twice a day—should have been enough, right? When she whined, I thought, *I don't want to get up. I have to do engineering.* She looked at me, and I told her, "*No.* Knock it off! Jesus, Obadiah, I have to concentrate!" So she'd know why she had to be quiet.

She made me nervous. I'd sweat instantly, but I couldn't let a drop fall on my paper. "Twice is enough!" I told her, to calm her down.

What they found in my notebook about cutting off my, my dick? That's just getting it out of my system. This, this was about not hurting my *dog.* It's more important.

Well, okay, I hate myself sometimes. It's not a big deal. That picture, the cutting, that's just me being screwed up from a long time ago. You'll see. I'm not a bad guy anymore. Just wait. You'll see.

I would forget what time it was, how long I'd been working, so she'd whine, and I'd look up—but I remembered all my assignments for the week. Then I'd stare at the shelf, to ignore her. Count my soups: one, two, three, one, two, three . . . one, two, *three,* one, two, *three,* one, two—

I know—*three*—sometimes I do that—I'll concentrate—one, two, *three*—

I'd count like that for ten minutes or so, get no work done. Because of the damn dog, and later I'd find pee, right there. Or she'd go to the corner but get up like ten or fifty minutes later and whine again. I'd say, "Stop!" and explain, and sweat again. Get mad and move something, then have to move all my books out of place and back into place. Restack my papers, settle in.

I would never get those minutes back—I hurt my teeth, chomp-chomping on each other—and I'd be mad even if she was sleeping. Took my 8H pencils—expensive ones—and used my X-Acto knife to sharpen them, sand the fucking points—I *am* calm—and blow away all that wasted graphite, and it went under the metal edge and turned that gummy stuff black so I'd have to rub along the edge, to mix it in perfectly. Then wash my fingers, under my nails. Waste *more* time.

Sometimes, I'd move the graphite around with one finger, make a row, a pile, a row again, and think how much new pencils cost. And cry.

Have to wash my fingers and clean up *again,* so my paper wouldn't—

I'd be so mad at Obie. Or sad. I'd say: "Please, *please*!" over and over, pull my hair, slap my—grab my face, real tight—

I know it was my fault, now. I thought I had to learn to *ignore* her—crazy, right? You can't say it, but I can.

～

Things got better when I learned to hook her up to the old swing-set out back, from when it was a real house. I didn't before, because why have a dog then? But I decided it was okay for lunch or when I went to morning classes.

But I hated how sad she was, all alone. Sometimes I changed my mind, as a treat, and took her back upstairs.

But if she peed—those sticky yellow puddles—even though I walked her in the morning—I'd get—I tightened my whole face and shoulders so I wouldn't hit her. Grabbed her by her collar and told her, "Bad dog." I hissed, like that. Stomped down the back stairs, hooked her up. She whined, but I told her, *Be a good dog*—in a friendly-but-still-mad way—and went back upstairs. To have my soup. Do my work.

If she *didn't* pee, I'd play with her out there. Pat her, act friendly the whole time.

Hooked-up was like going for a walk, but it still wasn't enough. This was almost—it was last year. I thought twice a day was enough, and it was important to teach her that. I couldn't let her *make* me walk her. I was training her. I'd stand over her until she stopped whining, then pat her. She let me think she learned it, too, the way she acted and all. Wanted to make me think that.

Almost always, by the time I went out to get her, I loved her again. She was so happy to see me, jumping all over, it was like a new morning. Everyone could see we loved each other, how I was a good guy with a good dog and all.

I know. God, it's—I *know* when I *cry*. I'm not mad. Just stop asking me if I can feel it.

I don't need a break. We're almost to the bad part that's the good part.

I asked her, "Why are you like this?" and "Why are you so God. Damn. Stupid?" I hated her at the exact second I loved her. Sometimes, I just hated her, to tell the truth. Forgot to love her at all.

⟨⟩

I was working. She didn't whine—at least I don't think so— and then I heard her pee by the door. I jammed my good pencil down, and the point broke. The point just snapped off in that rubbery old linoleum. A little circle of graphite with a swollen ring around it. A waste—all the lines and letters I could have made with that pencil point—never get it back—

I got up and stomped over. She tried to run, but I grabbed her by the collar—*some* of her neck—dragged her to where the towels were. She whined, she was scared, but I didn't care, she had to learn, Goddamnit—and I dragged her back, switched hands—grabbed fur, a bad—I'm *so sorry*, Obie. So I took just her collar, clenched really tight, *too* tight, all the way up my arm, in my shoulder, my face—

But I didn't hit her.

I wiped and wiped all that pee and made her smell the rag right on her nose. I said, "No!" and "Why?" and other stuff, mean stuff, *stupid* stuff, over and over.

I don't remember. I really don't. No. Okay, I do: Dad stuff. My real dad, before jail. Ancient history.

That was the only really bad time. She was afraid to run. I stood over her, made my face so tight I was dizzy, little gold and blue and black pinwheels—and I couldn't breathe. Like now, but a lot worse. I was so afraid I'd hit her, break her bones, her scrawny little neck, never stop hitting—like Dad.

Let me get to the end, okay?

I felt sick but also better, after that. I listened to her, and she did better. I came back from class and took her out back, when she wanted to. Walked her around outside before I took her in from the chain, stuff like that. Maybe I still wasn't walking her enough, I wasn't all-the-way thinking about *her*, see? I still wanted her to learn to not need so many walks.

Why didn't I take her out more, before, whenever she wanted? So stupid how I couldn't see it. Obie *told* me, told me *every day*, every time: "Take me out." But I wouldn't. I wanted to do my work, and I didn't see how she was my work, too. I loved Obie. Really loved her, not just pretend, for other people. I didn't hit her. I grabbed her hard on the fur that one time—I hurt her—I'm *so sorry*, Obie.

What? No, not forgivable. Never. I can't—but I didn't *hit* her. Not even that day.

I moved into the Vietnam Veterans Against the War house (though not a veteran), so I gave her away to some older students. One of them works in the library and made her a picture ID card, to hang around her neck. I see her with them, but she always goes crazy for me, jumps all over.

I wish I could go back in time, go up to that stupid boy, to me, and say: "Wake up!" I would explain to him: Dogs tell us what we need to know. She has to go when she has to go. I'd make him—*me*—understand: It wasn't personal. Don't know how I could get that into his head—my head, I mean. Probably have to take myself far away. Hold myself for, like, three days, rock myself, pat myself. Say, "Okay, okay" over and over, before I could even listen or learn anything. I was a stupid boy.

Now you think I'm a bad guy. I'm not. You have my notebook, all that old stuff from before, when I used to be a boy who wouldn't walk his dog. Now I know better. I *am* better. I don't think about anything that awful *ever*, not anymore. Almost never. And I talk to people now.

But I didn't—aren't you listening?—I *didn't* hurt myself. Didn't hurt anybody. I'm not like that, I'm not my dad.

To her? I'd say, "I'm sorry, Obie."

BEAUTY MARKS

RAE ALEXANDRA UNDERBERG

The first time I did it was out of desperation. There was no premeditation, just a blind groping for a solution to a problem that escaped my tongue. But the blood made the wordlessness less. Less frustrating, less infuriating, just less. I tried holding my hands together to steady them, clenching my jaw to keep the room from spinning. My chest burned, anger fired through my veins, bile crept up my throat. A ringing in my ears. Flashes of bright light. I shook my head, and it emptied. Darkness.

I started with scissors. They have a gray handle with yellow interior grips. I've had them since high school. I could try to make them romantic, imagine some attachment I have to these particular scissors, create some reason I've kept them for so long. But that would be a lie. I'm cheap, so I'm careful not to lose things. Most of the time I've spent using them has passed in frustration—at not being able to cut a straight line for a poster board or a circle without bulging tumors.

I held them open, pressed one blade against the pale inside of my forearm, and dragged it across the smooth skin. With enough pressure, I felt my skin slowly break away from itself, the cool metal edge drawing blood to the surface like a magnet. The pain wasn't really pain, because that would imply a negative, and it wasn't. It felt good. The separation, the coming to the surface, the release of pressure. The heat flooded in pinpricks across my face, down my shoulder, and over my forearm. I pressed down again. My eyes rolled upward; my heart slowed. The room dropped away behind me as the line of blood began to overflow from the valley and drip down my arm.

Again and again, I pressed down and slid the scissors across my arm until my hands shook. *Once*, I told myself. *Twice*, I told myself. *Three times*. But it wasn't enough. The scissors were inefficient, did not cut deep enough. And so I bought a box cutter. Sleek, black, silver. Ten turns of the screwdriver, and the blade was free. The blade so light, I barely felt its edge rest against my skin. But it was significantly better, pulling the layers apart effortlessly, as though it were made to slice skin, to draw blood.

When I press a tissue against fresh cuts, the blood spreads quickly. A drop becomes a splotch. A line grows in length and width into something larger, trying to take up space. I like the way it looks at first, the dark-red shapes and patterns against the white background. It could be a piece of contemporary art. When I'm finished, it looks overdone, like a child who receives praise for a scribbled drawing with the lines barely distinguishable.

In between each scab, I add a line. Peak, valley, peak, valley, peak, valley. The blood runs down between the mountains, a stream of life between the rocks. When the scabs heal, I make new lines above them, the highs and lows cycling, replacing each other. I'm surprised at how fast the liquid becomes solid, the blood clotting, sealing the exposed flesh.

I have small dark-brown beauty marks across my body. Not so many that they're prominent, but enough that they're noticeable if you really look. I've always liked the little dots. As a child, I used to connect them with pen to make pictures on my skin. One night with the blade, I noticed a dot in my path and decided to avoid it. Vanity in the face of disfigurement. But of course, vanity stood no real chance. A scab rests over the beauty mark now. I wonder if it will be there when the skin repairs itself.

I started cutting not long after college. That was three years ago, and I'm now a full-time case manager at a nonprofit in Brooklyn. I've since done plenty of research. I like to think I'm curious, but it's more of a selfish tendency that drives my wonderment, turning it malignant. I hunger for information, thirst for an explanation, chase what I can't understand until exhaustion overtakes me.

There are no accurate statistics about self-harm. Yes, there are studies that list the prevalence among specific groups of adolescents, but I question their accuracy. I hide the evidence from myself. Long sleeves that hide spots. Stained tissues folded into cleanliness. The fact of a survey doesn't inherently make the results true. People lie on paper, to strangers, to loved ones, to themselves.

My body craves it now as I write, legs shaking under the desk trying to run away from myself, to avoid confrontation, to quiet the internal voice badgering me. I tell myself I'm too old for this, that I was resilient before and nothing has changed, that there is nothing so bad in my life, no excuse to be unhappy. And then I ask myself why I didn't realize this before, why I like it so much.

According to the Mayo Clinic's website, self-harm is "the act of deliberately harming the surface of your own body" and that "while it may bring a momentary sense of calm and release of tension, it's usually followed by guilt and shame and the return of painful emotions." It's the solution to a problem that becomes, in its own right, a problem. The exposed skin that pulls farther apart with each movement, the scabs that threaten to open when snagged on a sleeve, the scars left behind marking brokenness.

Sometimes when I smile, I break away from the moment and ask myself, *Why can't you always feel this way?* The voice is angry but pleading—it's easy enough to be happy. But when the razor is in my hand, I don't have to shake the world away. I don't have a voice in my head. There is only the moment, the sensation that I can live here, just like this, forever.

⟾

Two-and-a-half years ago, when my sleeve slipped down in bed, I burrowed my head under the covers. But my boyfriend pulled me up. In almost four years together, I had never hidden anything from him before. But for three cold winter months after graduating college, the long distance made lying easy. Oversized sweaters; old, baggy long-sleeved shirts. A newly developed shyness and apprehension attributed to graduation and transition.

But now, my skin was exposed. The thin red lines streaked across my floral duvet had an origin. The balled-up tissues without a cold had an explanation. The packets of gauze on the dresser for invented kitchen accidents took on a different purpose.

"Look at me. Look at me. Look at me." He kept saying it, as though repetition would make it happen.

I kept my eyes trained on the flashy Georgetown degree on my wall. The excessive dimensions and pretentious Latin inscription embarrassed me. But I was grateful for it then, my eyes tracing the black frame over and over, their crooked orientation the only reason it seemed to belong on my wall.

There is no hiding shame. But he didn't want to see my shame—he wanted me to see his pain. The tears streaking his cheeks. Snot dripping from his nose. The coming together of eyebrows. Sharp intakes of breath. Surprise, confusion, anger. My self-harm had suddenly become outwardly aggressive, and fear clouded his eyes. He couldn't touch my arm, could manage only euphemisms, dissonance, the sharper words trapped in his mouth. He saw only brokenness, instability, cracks running through what was once pristine.

Whenever I've been cutting, I wake fiendishly scratching at the wounds. Attacking the healing process, I hurt myself even in unconsciousness. No residual dreams are left, only the itching sensation of a scab drawing broken skin together.

There's a biological explanation for this feeling. The nerve fibers that communicate the "itch" sensation from my arm to my brain are firing as the skin from the edges of each cut slowly makes its way to the middle of the wound to fill the new gap. The contraction activates my nerves, my brain screaming at my hands to scratch.

But it's not all cells and nerves and biology. It's hedonism. Scratching has the potential to damage tissue and cause pain. But it feels like a reward to me—it stops the itch. The head rush of satisfaction I get from scratching outweighs the pain of tearing away the scabs. It's a sacrifice. I want the instant gratification, even if that makes it worse.

⤳

After my boyfriend found out, I called the Georgetown library, flustered. Only nine months after graduation, my student ID number should still have given me access to all the databases, but I was caught in an obnoxious feedback loop. From the alumni access page to the search engine to the journals, and then the article link redirected me right back to the alumni page to sign in and repeat the process. My call was also redirected, from one gentle-voiced woman behind a desk to another.

I took a deep breath between the calls. Another breath. Most glitches can be fixed. Other graduates trying to research their lives had probably already filed a complaint.

"No access, but there's a link to click right there under what I want." Repeat, try again. I could hear the frustration simmering under my voice, the polite words bubbling over. Her soft voice told me to wait, that she'd find where I was, reach across the

Internet and follow my search to see with her own eyes what was happening to me.

"Okay, here we are, the alumni page, ProQuest, and the keyword?" Her inflection rose. I could imagine her skinny fingers, pale from days spent inside, hovering over the keyboard, her eyes looking up over the rims of her glasses, as if I were standing at her desk.

My throat closed. I wanted to understand. I wanted to make myself different from the research. I was searching for an explanation for something that I was ashamed to tell this gentle-voiced woman miles away. She would never know what I looked like or what was important to me or even my name. She would only know the sound of my voice distorted by a telephone, the nervous high-pitched crackling through her headset.

"The keyword you're searching for?" More declarative this time, a hint of raised eyebrows. A millennial should know what *keyword* meant, she'd think.

"Dementia?" Someone else's voice emerged from my lips, lower and croaky. This seemed like a safer answer than *self-harm*, one I'd researched hundreds of times before.

The first link on the page opened to an article, as did the second and third. She sounded confused now at my inability to replicate my own problem. I scrolled quickly, looking for a sign that one of these articles would lead to the same bad search cycle. I clicked and refreshed.

"Number 12!" I nearly shouted in glee at finding the glitch. "The twelfth article on the list. Click it and see." Proof. There was no way to gain access; it led to the same feedback loop. Relief. The gentle voice told me to come in and use the library computers.

"Thank you." I hung up and stopped searching.

⟶

Self-harm as self-care. That sounds paradoxical. Self-harm as self-protection. Still too contradictory. Self-harm as anti-suicide. Seems illogical. Suicide is sometimes thought of as the ultimate manifestation of self-harm.

My heart rushes whenever the red lights on the platform begin flashing to announce the arrival of the next Metro train. When it's imminent, and I can see the light at the end of the tunnel growing, I leave myself and feel only the rush of displaced air the moment before the train blasts past me. I often have the impulse to step in front of it. Cold, hard metal. Blunt-force trauma. High speed, warm blood.

This is not a suicide plan. There are never notes sitting on my desk meant to explain away the doubts that would follow. It's a fleeting thought, an electrical impulse traveling from axon to dendrite, neuron to neuron. But these impulses traveling through my brain are draining, leaving my head light, my heart heavy. The cold metal blade doesn't have the capacity for blunt-force trauma, for crushing my bones beneath its weight. The strength of my hand pressing the blade against the skin dictates the release of blood beneath. The Royal College of Psychiatrists tells me I am statistically more likely to commit suicide. I am alarmed knowing it and frightened writing it.

Wean yourself off the blade, I tell myself. Impose a limit. Only five cuts. I run the blade over my skin slowly, drawing each cut out as long as possible. I touch the tip of the blade to my skin and slide it a centimeter at a time, letting the entire blade run through each part of the opening cut. I focus on applying equal pressure across the blunt edge of the blade. I space them evenly across the rough patch of skin below the crook of my elbow. The old pink scars deepen to red as the blood rushes to the surface. When there are five fresh lines, I begin again at the first. Small clots dot the red streak, blocking the blood from escaping. The blade slips past the semi-congealed blood and back between the freshly separated layers of skin.

Blood flows faster the second time. By the time I get to the last one, there are no clots to cut away; I just carve deeper into the messy wet blood. Five, ten, fifteen. Beads of blood force themselves through the spaces between, run down the sides of my arm.

I lie to myself, leave only evidence of my imposed limit.

Try again. Go for fifteen minutes. Check the clock, 44 minutes after the hour, wait until the 4 becomes a 5, satisfy the need for evenness. My hand moves quickly; the blade flashes as it passes back and forth through my skin. There is no pink scar tissue left. Breathe, turn, check the clock: :03. Already over time, but add two minutes to satisfy the need for evenness. Stop five minutes after the hour.

Clean the blade, screw it back into the plastic box-cutter case, replace it in the desk. Clean the cuts, tape a bandage over the mess. Lie to myself.

I wasn't completely sober when I told my brother last year, but I wasn't drunk, either. It had been a long night, and when we walked into the apartment, I followed him into his room and sat in the red chair, the nap chair, my place in his room in our childhood apartment. He knew I was upset on the train ride home, not just because I'd fought with my boyfriend.

I didn't want to implicate him in my story, but I knew I had to tell my brother. I had moved back to New York, and it was only a matter of time before he accidentally saw my sleeves rolled up doing dishes or he saw my sleeve fall away from my wrist when I reached for something. I'd been anticipating this moment for months, playing the scene over and over in my head. Shock prying his eyes wide open, and then sadness bringing his lids back down. The way he'd immediately pull me into a hug, no questions asked, his wiry arms wrapped tight around my back, my head resting heavily on his chest.

He hasn't cried in years, but he might cry silently. I'd know only from the staggered breathing shaking his body, the hot tears hitting my back. We'd stand there for a few minutes, uncomfortable in the silence, but comfortable in our hug. And then he would sit me down and get serious, tell me we would fix it together, like we've always fixed everything.

Five in the morning was as good a time as any, so I unbuttoned my sleeve. But I didn't roll it up. I was desensitized to the red lines, but for him, it would be horrifying if I didn't say something first. My neck strained from keeping my head tilted downward. Tears blurred my eyes.

"Sometimes, I have to cut myself." I pushed the words from my mouth before they would be trapped, rotting in my gut forever. I didn't want to see his reaction.

Slipping down to the floor from his bed, he told me it was okay. His hand felt cold against my chin as he raised my face to look into his. I pulled away, and he made excuses for me: It was a hard year. He tried to normalize my destructive behavior, telling me what I already knew: He used to drink too much to make himself feel better. And then he rationalized for me: If I told him about it, I probably wanted to stop. He told me what I needed to do: Take three months and see if I could stop myself, and if I couldn't, then we would see about getting help. Until then, we wouldn't have to talk about it.

Curled up on the futon in the old room we shared growing up, I felt relieved. We didn't have to talk; he believed I could fix myself. The silence he created felt like a cushion to rest on, to hide under, to brace my fall. And then suddenly, the silence expanded around me. Out of control, filling the room, it suffocated me. I thought only about the alcohol being absorbed through my stomach and small intestine, coursing through my veins, thinning my blood. It would flow free and easy now, like warm water washing over my arms. The blade called. And then I felt alone.

～

When my first roommates after college created a burn narrative about the bandage I needed when the bleeding wouldn't stop, I let them tell their own kitchen-burn stories. I violated their trust, as they wholeheartedly embraced the lie, telling me about their lives, assuming they knew details about mine. When I bled through my long-sleeve shirts at the gym, I abused the kindness of strangers and let people tell me to watch out for rusty equipment because it stains. It's easier to lie by omission than try to explain the truth.

I hate being stared at. When I wear a T-shirt to the gym, it's not a cry for help. I feel hot and sweaty. And yet, I can't help myself from staring at others. My eyes linger on the woman on the elliptical who I believe has anorexia. I want only to look her in the eyes, put a hand on her shoulder, and tell her that I understand. Not what she is going through, but only that I understand pain, that I, too, have suffered and felt alone.

I flash back to the dining room in my first house after college, my neighbor joking that he's going to cut his wrists because of some frustration at work. His laughter, my silence. I flash back to our housewarming that same year. A guest saying she would kill herself if she didn't get into med school. Friends' sighs of sympathy, my silence. My shame.

⟶

Two years ago, I walked up the steps of a local tattoo shop in D.C. with a script in mind for explaining the scars and my idea in a few quick sentences. I'd picked a small place, figuring the need for business would overcome the instinct to ask questions. But as soon as the big-bearded artist towered over me, his bald head covered in tattoos, I stuttered. I didn't think he'd agree to do it.

My idea was vague, less an idea than a cloud of images and philosophy waiting to take form. The explanation flooded from my lips, muddled with the sweat of nervousness. The scars, slightly raised, were pale pink, still healing, stitching themselves together beneath the surface of my forearm. He met my confusion, the public display of private pain, with a raised eyebrow, inquisitive but also communicating pity. But he agreed, and I tried to pretend I didn't care what he thought of me.

The process felt good two months later, especially after abstaining to ensure the scars would fade and heal enough to take the ink. The pain of the needle was familiar, a welcome sensation after the hiatus the artist had imposed. The fast, sharp penetration of the skin over and over, breaking through the scar tissue, calling blood to the surface—relief flooding through my veins and skin.

I've had this tattoo now for more than a year. Two swooping black brush strokes form a circle around the scars, and in the center are the two Japanese characters for *wabi sabi*. If nosy strangers ask about it, I never mention the origin of the art, only explain that the symbols represent finding beauty in imperfection, incompleteness, impermanence. But *wabi sabi* also represents the recognition of two sides in everything. Stillness can be panic-inducing—but in darkness, there can also be calm. It's a constant reminder that everything I experience, everything I am and ever will be, is imperfect, incomplete, impermanent.

So, whenever the desperation builds and my world demands silence, my fingers find the blade. Blood drips around the tattoo, spreading from the center of my forearm nearer to the crook of my elbow and down closer to my wrist. The red lines are an important reminder, too.

Sources

"Self-Injury/Cutting," retrieved from the Mayo Clinic website (December 2015).

"Self-harm" by Keren Skegg, *The Lancet*, 2005.

"Self-harm" by Philip Timms, website of the Royal College of Psychiatrists, 2016.

"Wabi Sabi—Learning to See the Invisible" by Tim Wong and Akiko Hirano, *Touching Stone: Japanese Aesthetics in the Southwest*, 2016.

SPRING HARBOR, AGAIN

~~~

KRISTINE SNOW MILLARD

This time, the problem was pills. I hadn't yet swallowed the handful of Ativan tablets I'd counted out in my damp palm. I hadn't closed my eyes and counted to five while I drove down Deering Avenue. I hadn't sliced open my forearm with my secret piece of broken porcelain. I'd simply held the pills gently and imagined disappearing. But that was enough.

I walked through the shining double doors of Portland's Maine Medical Center and told the ER docs the truth: I want to kill myself.

I believe this happened at the end of 2004, although I was hospitalized several times during this period, and I've lost track of exact dates. I stretched out on a narrow bed in the psych department, answered obligatory intake questions—"Did something happen to make you feel this way?"—and waited for updates on the status of a bed at Spring Harbor Hospital, Maine Med's inpatient psychiatric facility. For nearly a dozen hours, under the watchful eye of a patrolling security guard, I waited, too desperate to think of excuses to sign myself out. Then two EMTs picked up my belongings in the blue hospital-issued plastic bag, rolled me into the cold December night, and once again took me away from Seamus and the girls. (I've changed their names and others here.)

Even more than death, I craved distraction. On the three a.m. ambulance ride down Congress Street, I played one of my favorite childhood car games. Without looking, I tried to place exactly where we were on the route to our destination. Thirty years earlier in New Hampshire, my younger sister Julie and I had entertained ourselves the same way. We would close our eyes in the back seat of Mom's Plymouth station wagon and guess our location on the narrow roads leading from the rectory in Durham to our camp at Squam Lake. Left out of Park Court, a few miles to the Spaulding Turnpike; then, 45 minutes later, winding roads through Alton and Gilford and Weirs Beach. We usually gave up long before we reached Meredith and Center Harbor and, finally, Holderness.

At 41, I was doing the same thing. But this time, I left my eyes open; I was strapped to a stretcher with just a tiny view of the black night outside the ambulance's back window. The game was a numbing diversion from the anxiety I felt about yet another stint in what I called "the clink." Down the hill by the dreary Greyhound bus station, then right on St. John Street— past McDonald's on the left, Dunkin Donuts and Sullivan Tire on the right. Left under the railroad bridge, then a straight shot out Congress Street. A few traffic lights, past Westgate Plaza, with the Shaw's supermarket that sold questionable produce and overpriced milk.

The EMT riding in the back with me was young. That's all I remember. That and brown hair. And a uniform. But I have no idea what color his eyes were, or if he had freckles, or whether he smelled good. He sat right next to me, near my head.

While I silently tracked our location on the rumbling ten-minute drive, he made small talk: Did I work, have kids, like to ski? Then he paused.

"You ever think about what would happen if you did it?" he asked.

At first, I was confused. *It*? I shifted under the white cotton blanket. Stroudwater Street. We were slowing down for the light, just past the bridge that crosses a marshy little inlet of the Fore River.

"I mean, I don't know if there's a hell or not," he said. "I just don't know if I'd want to take any chances."

He looked at me, held my gaze. When I'd told the ER doctor the previous afternoon that I felt like killing myself, I never thought about hell. What kind of believer was I with no hell factored into the equation? My Episcopal-priest father had never talked about hell, not at home or from the pulpit. But I was Catholic now, had converted to my husband's faith six years earlier, and yet, the afterlife hadn't occurred to me. I wondered if the ambulance crew was even supposed to talk about this stuff with patients.

Maybe he had a point about hell. Maybe there was torture out there, torture worse than the one I'd felt at home earlier while cupping the pills in my hand and calculating how many would make me sleep and sleep and sleep—and then wake up so that

Seamus would stop worrying, and Grace and Olive wouldn't be without a mother. Would there be fire and brimstone in hell, the kind you hear about as a kid? I didn't know what brimstone was. Was that normal, hearing a word a zillion times and never bothering to look it up? And the devil? All I could picture were those cheap red Halloween costumes with horns and a pitchfork, the ones they sold at the discount department stores my parents had hated.

I felt the ambulance bear right to stay on Congress Street just before the enormous UNUM insurance company building. I wished we could detour past the mall's calm parking lots, where years later we'd take our two daughters on Sunday nights to learn how to drive. We had already traveled as a family down this same road. The four of us rode in our clunky Volvo wagon to those remote dusty fields in Buxton for Sunday-afternoon youth soccer games. The girls were on travel teams, played years of weekend games from the end of August to late October. I went to each one of those games, sat next to Seamus in a collapsible nylon chair, and drank coffee from a travel mug while Bert, our labradoodle puppy, slept in the dusty grass.

Years later, when Olive had graduated from that Portland league and started on varsity as a high school freshman—when our arguments had escalated from verbal snipes to cruel, attacking words—she would tell me it didn't matter that I'd never missed a game. "You were so drugged out, Mom. It's not like you were *really* there." She was right. The antidepressants and mood stabilizers and tranquilizers my pharmacology-happy psychiatrist had prescribed—at one point, eighteen pills a day—took everything but my body away from the parenting equation. Those days, as a mother, I was null and void.

Maybe I should have been grateful for the nice EMT's question. In all the times I'd thought about suicide, it had never occurred to me that death might actually be worse than life.

⌒

A couple more traffic lights, then a right turn. Spring Harbor was only a few hundred yards away. My heart thumped, and I had to pee. During this part of the ride—every single time—I silently tallied the reasons I didn't need to be there. Seamus might have trouble getting the girls to bed. I just needed a med tweak. Other people went to Spring Harbor, the ones who slashed deep enough to need stitches, the ones found overdosed and unconscious across their beds. Other people wondered whether those last moments before death would bring fear or relief. I just struggled a little with depression and only occasionally admitted I had irrational thoughts. I wasn't unstable or unbalanced or *truly* at risk, not like the other patients. Was I?

Of course I was.

The ambulance slowed, rounded a corner, and parked at the back of the yellow building. I knew from previous stays—after the doctors had deemed me safe and discharged me during daylight hours—that the hospital was pretty enough from the outside to be a high-end condo complex or a retirement community. The EMTs opened the back door, pulled me out, then rolled me the short distance to the wide glass doors that opened automatically.

The inside of the building hadn't changed. Here, it looked like a hospital, with muted colors and mail-order artwork on the walls.

The ambulance driver—she had a brassy ponytail and too-snug pants—picked up my plastic bag of clothes. I'd arrived at the ER prepared: jeans, but no belts; clogs, because they didn't allow shoelaces. The hospital would be a perfect place to knit, but, of course, that wasn't allowed, either. I had a book and my journal; the desk nurse would lend me a stubby pencil from a box on her desk. I'd left my contacts and makeup at home. Still, I would shower every morning, no matter what. I might be on a locked unit. I might be checked for safety and monitored round the clock, but at least I would have clean hair. I had to have something going for me.

It felt good to walk, even the short distance from the stretcher to the intake room. I knew the drill: Someone would carry my stuff up to the unit. A psych tech would go through each and every item, looking for dangerous sharps. I couldn't even keep my own pen to write down how homesick I was about to feel.

"Kris?"

The staff member who walked into the room was William, from our old neighborhood. His kids went to the independent school where Seamus taught. His wife was a social worker, and they lived down the street from the school. Their son, the youngest of their three kids, was a grade below Grace. I could still picture him from a decade earlier, a three-year-old whizzing by on his tiny bike. Back then, mental illness had been a vague and generic term. It had applied to people without faces. It most definitely did not apply to me. I'd had no idea William worked at Spring Harbor.

"How are you, Kris?"

He met my eyes, saying without saying, *I know you, and you know me; maybe that will make this a little more bearable.* He was a pro; he didn't ask about Seamus's teaching or our girls.

"We need to ask you some questions before we take you up," he said. "We also need to take your picture for your chart."

Really?

Then I laughed to myself. Half a day ago, I hadn't wanted to live, and now, just for an instant, I cared about how I looked. But I didn't smile when William left and a woman materialized, holding a bulky camera in front of me. I didn't care that the instant photo taped to my chart would reveal a dirty-blonde bedhead, a pale face, and small, red, tired eyes behind thick glasses usually reserved for nighttime at home. I surrendered.

Then it was time for the security wand. As I spread my arms and legs, I wondered if they ever did strip searches. The woman waved the black-and-yellow paddle up and down, back and forth. I passed the test and sat back down in my corner seat. William had left the room, and now the woman—she hadn't told me her name—took the wand back to the office and returned with a clipboard and sheaf of white papers.

I wondered if William ordinarily did this part of the process. Maybe he'd turned the task over because he knew me. It had happened before—Portland is a small town. During one of my previous ER visits, the attending psychiatrist was the father of one of Grace's friends; we'd had brunch at their apartment a few years back. I had told a nurse I didn't want him to evaluate me, so she sent in a resident instead. Of course, if it had been a physical injury, a broken bone or a bagel-cutting accident, knowing the doctor on call would have been fine, even preferable. Had I been embarrassed that night or ashamed? Do patients perpetuate the stigma of mental illness or just resign themselves to it? A bit of both?

"Just a few questions, Kristine." The woman smiled, sitting on the loveseat across from me. The litany began: What did I do for work, and did I have a therapist, and the famous "What brought you to the hospital"? If I were lucky, I'd die from tedium.

⤙⟶

Twenty minutes later, we rode the elevator in silence to the second floor. I had relinquished my watch in the ER, but guessed it was close to four a.m. I'd barely slept during my twelve hours at Maine Med. Now, I plodded behind my escort. I wanted only to change into hospital scrubs and climb into bed.

One of the nurses behind the horseshoe-shaped station walked toward us.

"Hi, Kristine," she said. "We'll go through your bag, and then you can have it back, okay? Let's just get your vitals, and you can get some sleep."

I dutifully walked over to the chair she'd pointed to and sat down. A wave of homesickness swept over me. Two days, I decided. I would stay for two days, max, and then I'd tell them I was better. Yes, I could do this for two days.

The long hallway to my left was quiet, its lights dim. From where I sat, I could see the first few rooms on each side of the corridor. Their doors were ajar, open just enough for the psych techs on duty to look in every fifteen minutes. Being locked on a unit and under constant supervision was reassuring in a way that told me how much I needed to be there. When I began to feel suffocated, began to yearn for the freedom of home, I'd know the crisis was over. But as I sat there with the thermometer under my tongue, waiting for the blood pressure monitor to finish beeping, I felt relieved. I was at Spring Harbor. Maybe, again, I'd proved all by myself how sick I really was.

FAMILY

I went back to your bedroom. You weren't breathing. I answered the questions. Alcohol. Drugs. Addict. Heroin. Hepatitis-C. You were on the floor. I held you on the floor. I put my cheek against your cheek. Your mouth was open. You had perfect teeth. My teeth are ugly.

—Drew Ciccolo

STORMS OF THE CIRCUS WORLD

LORRI McDOLE

Lightning

We never know what the weather will be, but every Labor Day weekend, my family vacations at a rustic resort on Orcas Island, located in the northwestern corner of Washington state. This evening, we build a fire on the beach, betting that the rain is at least an hour away. While my husband goes next door to the country store for marshmallows, my dad and I line up chocolate and graham crackers. My children, ages seven and ten, watch my brother sharpen branches into roasting sticks, the taste of burnt sugar already on their tongues.

Suddenly, my brother stops whittling.

I hope you know, he says, working a cigarette to the side of his mouth and looking into my children's faces, *that the only thing wrong with drugs are the narcs and the collectors.*

And just like that, the storm is on us.

The First Long Driveway

My brother ran away every day the year he was two. Mom would settle in to nurse our baby sister, and he'd slip out the screen door, kicking up gravel as he ran down our driveway. Caught between loyalty and obedience, I'd watch until he seemed in danger of disappearing altogether before running to tell her: *Randy gone.*

I don't really remember—I wasn't quite four—and yet this is the oldest memory my brother and I share, sewn into our psyches by Mom's stories. My brother, the would-be escape artist, and me, his reluctant savior.

Gathering Dark

When Randy and our cousin Steve were fourteen, they pushed a raft of stolen dynamite out into the middle of Plummer Lake in Centralia, Washington, our hometown. The explosion blew out the windows of several lake houses, racking up $3,000 in damages, a $500 fine, and several days in juvie for both boys. Because my brother was a few months older than Steve, everyone in our extended family blamed him.

A few years later, Steve was out with a school friend and drunk-drove his Jeep into a tree. Both boys died flying through the windshield.

When Randy heard that Steve's shoes were found on the floorboard of the car, as they often are in accidents, he collapsed into Dad's arms. *They should have been my shoes*, he sobbed. *It should have been me.*

An Idea

Your son is doing drugs, Mom said to Dad.
Hush, Nancy, you'll put ideas in his head.
She pointed to the dirty ashtray in Randy's bathroom.
There's an idea for you.

What Randy's Good At

Taking care of pets, hunting wild game, building things with his hands, gardening, telling stories. *I rode shotgun! The biggest gun in the West! I bet you didn't know there was such a gun, but I'm here to tell you: There is!* My sister tries to bring him down after one sentence—we've got to keep him in this world, she says—but I am mesmerized, surfing the ledge with him while he weaves his singular metaphors through our shared, storied landscape.

A Clue

One clear fall day when we were teenagers, I found my brother standing in the front yard, holding a leaf and staring up at the sky.
What are you doing? I asked.
Wondering how I ended up here.
In the yard?
In the world. In the world yard. Everyone thinks there's a million yards in the world, but maybe it's the other way around.

But no matter how anyone looks at it, we still don't have a clear idea: Which came first, the drugs or the schizophrenia?

A Mystery

Randy used to run with a boy who was later found on the Fords Prairie railroad tracks in Centralia with his arms and legs tied behind him, a deal-gone-bad bullet to the brain.

Questions of grief over my brother's wasted life—*why him? why us?*—changed for a time to guilty relief. At least he didn't do it. At least he wasn't the one on the tracks.

But soon enough, we were back to the questions: How can a person gunning so hard for himself dodge so many bullets?

The Big List, Alphabetically Speaking

- acid
- alcohol
- car wrecks (four?)
- children he barely knows (three)
- cigarettes
- cocaine
- Dad's charred bedroom
- death threats (received and delivered)
- ex-girlfriend's restraining order
- fights (three facial bones broken and hearing ruined in his right ear)
- glue
- halfway houses and the state hospital (five extended stays between them)
- jail (several stints)

- knife slashes and bullet grazes (some inflicted by other people)
- leaps from the roofs of trucks and houses (broken and sprained ankles)
- Lithium (when he takes it)
- middle-of-the-night lurches (countless) down the hall while Dad tried to hold him up
- middle-of-the-night pleas (countless): *Don't tell my sisters. Please don't tell my sisters.*
- Mom's finger-bruised neck
- mushrooms
- overdoses (stomach pumped twice)
- pot
- psychiatrists (three)
- schizophrenia (we finally figured out)
- things I don't know
- what I will never tell

Why Randy Lives with Dad

The government has stolen his money, millions they first denied taking and have now misplaced. He's too weak to leave, but after he stockpiles enough protein drinks (260 cans bought with his disability pay, and counting), he'll be ready. A lot of women want to marry him, their disembodied voices whispering relentlessly in his good ear, but he can't choose.

Occasionally, Randy makes it to the *T* of Dad's long gravel driveway, but then the government scrambles his internal GPS, and he doesn't know which way to turn.

Why He Really Lives with Dad

We've tried a few halfway houses and sent him through the state hospital system, but they were temporary fixes to a permanent problem. Besides, despite well-meaning clamors from all sides over the years for Dad to kick Randy out, a tough-love pill that treats mental illness has yet to be invented.

What I Don't Sleep About

Thirty years ago, when Dad asked me to bail Randy out of jail with my college money, I refused with a clear conscience.

What will I say now if he asks me to take Randy in when the time comes? Now that Mom has died and Dad is 78, when we have to sell Dad's house to pay off the mortgages, where will my brother go?

Nothing is clear anymore.

Listen

The man on this page is the man my brother became, but this man is not my brother. My brother couldn't pass me in the hall without kissing me on the cheek and thought I looked like every princess he saw on TV. My brother always invited me to play baseball with his friends, even though I sucked, and he once slammed the door on a friend who asked him to take the blanket off me while I was watching TV in my nightgown. My brother heard tires screech in the night and went out with soap and water to scrub what was left of our cat off the road so the rest of us wouldn't have to see it in the morning.

Confession

That time up on Orcas Island, after Randy told our kids about the narcs and collectors—but before my husband and I made the ultimatum that banned him from our trips for several years—I watched him stretch out over the end of the dock to pull up one of his makeshift crab pots. He lay there forever, it seemed, and I fantasized about him not getting up. I imagined him sliding, seal-like, beneath the surface, while I just watched him go without saying a word.

In a Boat in the Circus of the World

After four months of excruciating pain and endless tests, Dad has been diagnosed with a "non-specific virus." Gone is his part-time job and his ability to drive and cook. He can't cut up food, write out checks, clip his nails, zip his pants.

As a Christian, he believes it's wrong to take a life, even if it's his own. But on the nights he can walk, he paces, crying and rubbing his hands, not sure he can live like this.

While my sister and I run around in the background, handling insurance and the VA, paying bills out of Dad's social security and wringing *our* hands, my brother trims Dad's beard and hair and nails. He mows the acre of grass and keeps the fire going all night so the house is never cold. He empties the bedpan, lifts Dad into the bathtub, makes and feeds him dinner, times all medicines to the minute, and collaborates with the visiting nurses about how to get Dad to gain weight.

I haven't been trained on how to run budgets, he says nervously on the phone one day, *but I know that one less bottle of beer for me is one more can of Instant Breakfast for Dad. Every time I'm at the store, my brain gets exercised with the calisthenics of calculation!*

The last time we visited from Seattle, my sister went straight in to Dad, while I stopped on the porch with Randy. I made small talk, wondering anxiously which topic, or planet, we'd land on. He sat quietly for several minutes, courteously blowing his cigarette smoke away from me, and then jumped up.

Did I ever tell you about the first time I gave Dad a shower?

Uh-oh, I thought, where's *this* going? I shook my head.

I tried to get him to wait. The visiting nurse was going to be here any minute, but Dad didn't want to be dirty when she got here. I was like, well, Dad, what are you going to do, marry her?

He gave a nervous giggle, his voice revving low before vibrating to a higher octave: not the laugh you'd expect from a six-foot-two bearded man in a plaid quilted jacket. *But he was bound and determined, and I couldn't figure out how to help him except to get in with him, clothes and all. And Dad goes, well, Randy, you're getting all wet! And I go, well, Dad, so are you!*

We were both near tears then, laughing.

By the time the nurse got here, we were done and dry, and then in Dad goes again with her. Only she stayed outside the shower—this isn't that kind of story. He giggled again. *Anyway, now we've got it down. But that first time, it was like we were in the same boat! Which, of course, we've been in the same boat all these years. But now, well, now it's different, since I'm steering.*

I wondered if he was thinking about all the times Dad had guided him down the hall at 3:00 a.m., back before Mom got fed up with everything and left Dad to do everything alone. But all I said was, *Steering* and *rowing.*

Randy startled. *I guess you're right! You always were the smart one. But I must be doing okay, because we haven't done any capsizing that I know of. Of course, we don't talk about it. We just keep traveling around in this same boat, going in circles, our own little circus. It's something else, this circus of a world. I've seen a lot of things, and I'm telling you, I've never seen a damn thing like it.*

LOCKED DOORS

AMY McVAY ABBOTT

The hospital was as I remembered—anemic green walls, dingy white-tile floors. I took the steps two at a time, hurrying to my mother's room on the second floor. Dad was not far behind me, parking the truck.

Twelve hours earlier, he'd called with the news that Mom had drunk Drano. My college friend picked me up at the Indianapolis airport in the darkest part of night. We met my father at my parents' house, then Dad and I drove on to the hospital. I had traveled all night from Tampa.

As Mom stared at me from her hospital bed, she looked unscathed. Was I expecting a tourniquet around her neck—bloody, scarred, visible wounds?

"I'm upset you're living with your boyfriend," she said.

No "hello" or "what are you doing here?" We lived 1,200 miles apart.

Seriously? Did I say that aloud? I'm not sure.

"Mom, did you drink poison?" I asked.

93

"Maybe I did," she said. "Maybe I wanted to. When your dad came home from school, he thought we should go to the Emergency Room, so here we are."

Yes, here we were. Mom told her story as if it had been rehearsed a dozen times. She also wasn't surprised I stood at the end of her bed. Earlier that week, we'd talked on the telephone. She knew I had received my $459 tax-return check and could afford to fly home. I wasn't surprised she was in the hospital.

⟜

Mom had been depressed and anxious for a long time, but it wasn't a topic of regular conversation. In the 1960s, an internist prescribed what we then called "nerve pills." Mom never stayed with those pills long; she said they made her sick to her stomach.

My mother was trained as an elementary school teacher with a reading specialty. She and my father, also a teacher, married in June 1955. In 1956, she lost her job as a second-grade teacher in Swayzee, Indiana, when her new pregnancy showed on her tiny frame. Absurd as it seems today, the swelling belly of a married woman in that small town was deemed a threat to school kids, but she never questioned her forced retirement at 24. She stayed at home with her children—a dutiful wife, a Sunday School teacher, a driver for us. She shared her passion for reading with my brother and me, Aesop's gory *Fables* along with poetry by Poe and Longfellow, Lear and Cummings.

And yet, both my mother and grandmother struggled with anxiety and depression, and, ultimately, dementia. Were the conditions related? Neither science nor I know for sure. In my family history, mental illness and dementia stand like bookends between generations. I've struggled with the twin demons of anxiety and depression for most of my adult life. Having witnessed how much can be lost, I take medication to stave off severe episodes.

My mother's illnesses resulted in several more inpatient stays until Prozac came out. Prozac was the first of the new drugs, without the baggage of the old pills. Mom started taking Prozac in the early 1990s and never had another hospitalization. She and I made peace after my son was born in 1990, a mutual truce for the rest of her life.

In 1971, when I was thirteen, a nearby church asked Mom to develop an early-reading curriculum for a new preschool. For weeks, she was a person I didn't know, carrying my grandfather's gnarly leather satchel to meetings. Only men took leather bags to business meetings. Women made punch, served in crystal cups with matching saucers for the literary society.

Mom dug out college textbooks and researched curriculum. She typed on a Smith-Corona electric typewriter, planning at the dining room table.

One summer evening, she met with the church board about funding. Mom wore a nice outfit—a turquoise skirt suit, dress heels, pearls, and matching clip-on earrings. Her wedding pearls and the white piping along the suit's lapels contrasted with her dark hair. At 38, she resembled Jackie Kennedy.

I was in my twin bed when she got home. With no air conditioning, our screened windows stayed open all summer, and I awakened when the garage door rose. Dad was sleeping in front of the TV set, *McCloud* blaring.

I heard Mom tell Dad she didn't get the job. Dad questioned her. He'd thought it was all sewn up. She said the board decided not to fund the preschool. The church needed a new roof, and two expensive projects weren't on the table.

She cried. Dad told her how sorry he was, and I suspect he put his arms around her. She must have put the satchel and papers away, because I never saw them again. She didn't talk about it with my brother and me. We were a tween and a teenager, with no clue our parents ever experienced disappointment.

But Mom was different after that. Or maybe I was different. I headed to the high school in September. I was mouthy and sure of myself as unsure teenagers are.

After her rejection by the local church, most evenings Mom dozed in her recliner with an *Ideals* magazine across her lap. My brother and I grew up, finding people and interests away from our parents. Mom spent her days with my grandparents and countless doctor's appointments and pharmacy runs. She dealt with a mother who had her own neuroses and a father with vascular dementia. To her parents, she was the perfect daughter.

Still, she said things out of context that made no sense. The furnace was poisoning her with gas fumes. Dad had it checked. She didn't accept the furnace man's verdict, so Dad bought a new furnace. Easier to make peace.

No one in our family or community spoke openly about mental illness. We whispered when a man shot himself in his barn. In a rural area of Indiana with plenty of guns, suicides were no surprise. Women didn't kill themselves as often. Some women took Valium or medicated with white wine—maybe too much Valium. Did the obituary in the weekly newspaper say "natural causes"? Probably.

When I was a small child, my mother was the best mother in the neighborhood, the one who played on the floor with us. She planned perfect birthday parties, read us amazing books, colored with us. Mom laughed and giggled and sang silly songs she made up, like, "Once I went in swimmin' where there were no wimmin' and no one to see—came a little bear, and stole my underwear, and left me with a . . . *SMILE*."

She wasn't like the other mothers. She was better. And then she wasn't.

The incident with the preschool job had burrowed into my memory, forgotten until her suicide attempt a dozen years later in 1983.

Dad found the two of us in Mom's hospital room, glaring at each other like prizefighters before a match. Did she drink the Drano? Was this a cry for help or a stand against me? Did I cause this? Was Mom triumphant in her assertion of my sin?

Her doctor came in and told us she needed more help than he could give. She would move to a psychiatric hospital in a nearby town, probably for a week or more. We could pick her up in the afternoon and drive her there.

The doctor left. Mom sat upright in the crank-up metal bed. Was she miserable or gleeful about the added attention? I couldn't tell. Dad told her we'd be back to take her to the hospital, then hustled me out of there as if we were late for the Lions Club Father-Daughter Banquet. I was grateful for our hasty exit.

In the truck, Dad said we were going to see his pastor. We drove into the country, where the brick church spire rose above ordinary farmhouses. The parsonage, a white, aluminum-sided two-story home, stood feet from the brick Lutheran sanctuary. The century-old congregation was a safe place for my family, and I understood Dad's desire to go there.

At the parsonage, Pastor and his wife greeted us. The couple invited us into the kitchen and served us coffee. The room was flooded with morning light, which annoyed me. I was tired and not ready for a presumed lecture on my spiritual shortcomings. My eyes roamed, noticing items out of place, a crèche on the dining room table, a Farm Bureau calendar turned to the wrong month.

The pastor's wife rested her elbows on the Formica kitchen table and twisted her gold wedding band. She talked about her own problems. Her forthrightness startled me. She confessed how frustrated she was when her life revolved around her husband's work and their five children. She admitted she battled depression, how occasionally she sought treatment.

I was speechless. This was the last place I thought I'd find clarity. A woman's place in the patriarchal German Lutheran community was firmly behind men. For her to share this intimacy with us was beyond amazing. We never talked about such personal details at the 150-year-old church where my parents had married. This woman laying open her wounds, admitting her fears and doubts, was Christianity at its finest.

Dad shared that Mom told me she'd tried to harm herself because she was upset I lived with my boyfriend. Pastor assured me I was not at fault, that my mom's issues had nothing to do with me. (He didn't bring up the boyfriend, although he married us a year later.) Pastor affirmed the doctor's recommendation that Mom needed inpatient treatment. He suggested I get counseling to work through my own guilt or grief.

We took Mom to the psychiatric hospital that afternoon in the beat-up blue truck. Dad and I were teary and uncertain. Mom was chipper and excited; she seemed almost glad. We drove west, past barren orchards and unplanted fields. The warm April day taunted us with a promise of early spring. Yet the twenty-minute drive seemed like three hours. I was afraid of what would happen to her at the hospital. What I knew about mental hospitals came from late-night movies, and it wasn't good.

The freestanding inpatient center was a stout cement-block building. An office behind a locked steel door led to a hidden room behind another locked door. A social worker met us in the first room, and Dad gave her the transfer papers.

"Say goodbye now," the social worker told my father. "You can't go behind this door."

We couldn't go in with her. We were expected to say goodbye right then, in the stark lobby, with no time to offer encouragement or extra hugs. Dad handed Mom her suitcase. The social worker swiped a white card on a lanyard against the front lock and told us that visiting hours were two to four on Sunday. She handed Dad a bundle of papers.

Mom kissed us both and moved back, as if she were getting on a bus to summer camp—*goodbye*—and we went through the locked front door.

I turned back to see the inner door open, Mom and the social worker stepping inside. Almost simultaneously, I heard the click of each latch, two steel doors locking behind us.

Two sharp clicks—a change in me. I knew it wasn't my fault. I knew Mom was ill.

My father, who had held it together the entire day, now sobbed. He wasn't a middle-aged teacher. He was a twelve-year-old boy in a haymow, listening as the sheriff took his mentally ill and violent older brother away from their farm. I helped Dad into the passenger side, and I drove the truck home.

The crazy thing about all this—the really crazy thing—is that once Dad was in the truck, once I was behind the wheel, everything was okay. We were dealing with reality rather than whispers or surface emotions. The truth, split open, forged the right path home.

WHAT IF

～

MADELEINE HOLMAN

I'm on the trail early to avoid the heat, but I'm soon covered in sweat. The path starts narrow and cave-like, with an overhang of limestone. It seems more expansive than usual, as if the canopy has been lifted. Still, I bend a little and lower my head to pass through, an old habit. The limestone wall muffles the sound of traffic on the busy road that runs parallel to the path. Farther on, where it's harder to ignore, the drone of passing cars competes with the incessant chirp of crickets.

It's June 2016, and soon I'll be seventy. As I make my way along the gravel path, I see other senior walkers, an animated, paired-up group. I could join them and not be alone. But I enjoy not having to talk.

Almost twenty years ago, I brought one of my sisters to this place, a favorite park of mine in Austin. My sister—I'll call her Jill, although that's not her name—used to walk for hours. But on that day, she was unsure of her footing, so we held hands as we had in childhood—I her older sister, but only by a year. We made our way from the limestone overhang to where the path was interrupted by the creek. It was late fall then, and there had been plenty of rain. It was chilly. The creek water rushed across boulders, forming a little waterfall just beyond the large flat rocks that people hopscotched on to get from one side of the creek to the other, where the path continued.

Jill was scared, her small frame swallowed up by an ill-fitting jacket. Even with glasses, her vision was poor. Long, uncombed hair fell across her face, further impeding her ability to navigate. I tried to encourage her to stay close so we could move together. The way across was clear, and there was no other option, but she stood still and wary. For a moment, I tried to convince her. "Hold onto my arm, I'll help you." But I soon realized my plan to share this fall afternoon with my sister had been wishful thinking.

Later, when outings with Jill took more energy than I could mobilize, the city built a concrete bridge across the creek. Children and dogs could still play in the shallow water on one side of the bridge, where smaller rocks remained. Cyclists no longer had to stop and lift their bikes to get across. My walk became seamless. No more hopscotching adventures for me, no more attempts to help Jill face insurmountable barriers.

Long ago, when we were both in our twenties, Jill drove to see me in Connecticut soon after graduating with honors from the art school at Tufts University in the Boston area. Our parents and other siblings were traveling abroad that summer. I was the only family around when she became increasingly unmoored. Day after day in my apartment, I found her circling, moving from stove to table, leaving a trail of colorful, undecipherable pictures, never eating. We were nervous together. Even when the bathtub overflowed, and I came home to find her in confusion and the landlady up in arms, I approached the situation as if it were only an accident.

My boyfriend and I looked at each other and found no way to be useful. We had no experience with madness. I spoke to Jill softly, aware of her fragility but afraid to name it. Was it drugs? A high that would run its course?

I made room for the art supplies she'd strewn around the apartment, part of a major project that never materialized. When I returned from work in the evening, she would be wandering again. Eyes wide open, she was entranced by all objects in her path: an ashtray carved to resemble an owl, a wooden spoon from Morocco, my grocery list, the canceled stamp on an envelope. "Are you sure you'll be okay?" I asked, when she stuck to the notion of driving cross-country in her blue Volkswagen bug.

This would become my mantra in the years to come—as would *if only*.

Jill made it only as far as Ohio, where police found her on the side of the road, her face and body smeared with paint of every color. Red, green, yellow, magenta—streaked through her long thick hair—a wild, tie-dyed disaster. She'd cut both wrists but was alive. The police used mace to force her out of the car.

During the next few years, I visited my sister at Fairfield Hills State Hospital, upstate in Newtown, Connecticut, where, after exhausting her insurance coverage at private facilities, Jill was admitted numerous times for psychotic episodes. Her diagnoses shifted between schizophrenia and schizoaffective disorder.

I have no memory of being at Fairfield Hills. I don't recall what the hospital looked like at that time, although I've since found pictures of its red-brick exterior; dingy white columns with peeling paint; rows of evenly spaced, long, narrow windows.

A few years ago, I saw more pictures of its abandoned corridors and cavernous rooms in a photo-essay book documenting the demise of abandoned state mental hospitals. I was part of a weekly study group that included psychiatrists, fellow therapists, and an architect, who passed this book around at one meeting for us to peruse. (I believe it was the 2012 volume *Beauty in Decay*.) We'd been exploring the relationship between architecture and psychoanalysis, and the architect presented images of decay in cities such as Detroit and at institutions like Fairfield Hills, which closed in 1995.

As I recall, the book was beautiful. It could sit prominently on any coffee table, if the subject weren't so bleak. I wanted to make the book uglier. I wanted to speak up about my family's intimate connection to what happened in those halls. "This is not art," I wanted to say. But instead, I flipped through a couple of pages and passed it along to the colleague next to me, hoping she wouldn't notice I'd fled the academic discussion I had found so stimulating just moments before. I didn't know these people well enough to make it personal.

⟿

In the late 1970s, my father retired and moved to Austin with my mother and Jill. Dad was born in Texas and had always wanted to go back one day. At the time, however, our family didn't know that Texas state mental hospitals were the focus of a 1974 lawsuit known as "RAJ," short for the name of a patient on whose behalf advocates sued the mental health department. The plaintiffs alleged rampant abuse and inadequate treatment. It took more than two decades for the state to meet minimum court-mandated treatment standards and for the lawsuit to be settled.

My father and I knew firsthand what bedlam was. I spent many weekends writing letters and articles decrying the neglect we witnessed. We met with legislators, demanding they attend to the abysmal hospital conditions and nonexistent community alternatives.

My mother died in 1988 after a long illness; my father died almost ten years later. After a painful divorce, I'd moved to Austin in the early eighties with my three-year-old daughter. At Dad's request, I became what's known in Texas as a "successor guardian" for Jill, since my other siblings lived far away and I was the oldest. When resentment stung, I channeled it into advocacy for Jill, meeting with her doctors and social workers, leading our National Alliance on Mental Illness (NAMI) chapter.

I went downtown for the guardianship hearing and stood before a judge who knew my family through myriad crises that involved the bench, including Jill's transfers from street to jail to hospital and court-ordered medication. The judge seemed sympathetic. He counseled me about what guardianship meant, but the responsibilities were not too different from what I was already doing. *I'm not a novice*, I wanted to shout at him, but instead I just said *yes*. I didn't want to risk offending him.

When I left the courthouse, I walked past an old church. Carved in stone above its side door was this motto: *Be Prepared*.

Now, hospital staff were supposed to notify me, as they had my father, about treatment or discharge planning. But I already knew there was no plan, no magic pill, no adequate community-based alternatives to the hospital.

⟜

Grief over our father's death was still raw, especially for Jill. Dad had been her anchor, always ready to support her. In addition, she was caught in the middle of a bad medication change. A week after Dad's funeral, she'd slugged a patient and several hospital staff.

I sat at the foot of a mattress on the floor of the seclusion room, while she lay curled up at the other end. Tiled walls; linoleum floor; a small, high window. The attendant left the door open. I read her a letter from one of our sisters, and it made me cry. Almost everything made me cry.

I read to her from a book of short stories I no longer recall. The stories weren't very interesting, but they gave me something to do. I would have read from them longer, if she hadn't put her hands over her ears.

A few months later, the nurse at the hospital echoed my observation that Jill had been "more present" lately. My sister Margaret was in Austin to help sort and divide up my parents' belongings. Margaret went to see Jill and took her to the canteen, where she was amused when another patient—a tall, broad-shouldered, middle-aged man—asked if Jill had finished her soda and grabbed it without waiting for an answer.

"We're not done," Margaret said, taking the can back just before it reached his lips.

Margaret told me: "Another guy there kept saying 'you look so different, you're so different,' over and over. He must have thought I was you."

I moved my parents' three-leaf dining table to my house. "You have the table," Jill said, when I brought her home on a pass. I reminded her about the family lore—*someday Mary will have this table and all its linens and chairs*—and how I could not imagine having someplace big enough to put all that. Jill nodded and smiled. She prepared part of her own dinner, combining feta cheese over noodles and tomato sauce, helping herself to a chocolate Ensure stacked with other canned goods from my father's kitchen.

I went through the stack of mail that had piled up at my parents' house. "Here's yours," I said, handing my sister her bank statement. There were several thousand dollars in her account. "Wow," she said.

⟨⟩

She was getting better. I could see it. The nurse and the psychiatrist saw it. At a treatment team meeting the next month, we sat around the table, smiling.

Jill sat beside me. She was doing her best to participate, staying put and not grimacing. She made eye contact and didn't mutter to herself. Going through the list of topics to be addressed—behavior, treatment plan, discharge outlook, medication—the nurse directed his words to Jill. We were all happy.

Before the meeting had started, Jill and I sat in the visitors' room, where I'd told her about my plans to go to graduate school to get a master's in counseling.

"I'm going to be broke," I said.

"I have money," she said, and I remembered how generous she'd been when I visited her in college long ago, when she was living with roommates and creating beautiful silkscreens and lithographs, cooking elaborate dinners, taking me under her wing as if she were the older sister.

⟨⟩

One evening in early summer, about six months after Dad's death, I walked Jill back to the hospital unit and pushed the buzzer. I told her I'd be away on vacation for several weeks. "I won't be able to see you for three weekends."

"Three weeks?" she said.

I wondered if my attention was partly responsible for her improvement, an attribution both seductive and oppressive. I thought of something I'd read in a book on Quaker history: The result is not the most important thing. *Right action is more imperative.* My father called it duty. Sometimes, the result we strive for never comes. But we still need to do the work, continue the action. I'd long ago abandoned the church liturgies I'd grown up with, but the silence of the Quaker meetings I attended often brought me solace and a sense of acceptance.

Right action is imperative. This is what I told myself then and later when, for months or years, Jill didn't respond to me, to coming home, to letters from our other sisters. Keep writing, keep visiting. At times, nothing seemed to matter. But I still went through the motions, continuing rituals of food or snacks and watching Kuma, my golden retriever, vie for Jill's and my attention.

I was veteran enough to be wary of Jill's new alertness. After all, the nurse had told me that several other patients were also improving after a long time in an environment where little changed. "I don't know what's happening this summer," he'd said.

And yet, I couldn't help fantasizing about what my life would be like if Jill really could take care of herself or had a network of support that would allow me to step aside. Could I consider out-of-state Ph.D. programs? Could I move closer to Margaret or join Catherine back in New England, which I still found myself missing every fall?

⟶

With a friend, I drove past several apartment complexes where people with mental illnesses lived in supported housing.

"Jill could have a peer companion," my friend said.

"Will that be enough?" I asked. "She has to take her meds, or she'll plummet again."

I looked into community programs like Gould Farm in Massachusetts, then dropped the idea. A woman had come to our NAMI meeting and shown a film about this community for the mentally disabled. When I asked about what was required of a resident like Jill, she said, "Your sister would have to be able to save herself in case of fire—to leave the building. She would have to make an effort, even if she couldn't perform her tasks at first."

Sometimes, Jill froze as I walked her back to the hospital unit after dinner. Sometimes, she'd freeze again at the door when the attendant ushered her in.

In the early 1990s, it had taken a long time to come back from her experience in a personal care home in East Austin, where the refrigerator was padlocked and the only air conditioning was in the staff's living quarters. Jill had been much improved prior to that move, but it turned out to be little more than a boarding house. She would get dizzy crossing the street to go to the 7-Eleven and tottered at the curb. Once again,

I had sat with her while she curled up in a corner and said, "I'm degenerating."

~

The cool weather I'd yearned for throughout the endless summer months finally arrived in October. I'd started grad school and was invigorated by taking on something new, just for me. Awakening in the night, I'd felt deeply comforted by the sound of heavy rain. Now, in the morning, the trees no longer stirred.

Combining errands and obligations, I loaded Kuma into my car and drove to the vet clinic, where she squirmed through her annual checkup. Procrastinating, I made one more stop before going to see how Jill was doing. If well enough, we could walk to the canteen for a snack. Having Kuma with us would provide an additional focus. And I had a bonus—a letter from our sister Catherine.

Jill looked like a kid, and, for a moment, I was startled. I caught a glimpse of my lost sister, with short curls framing her face, a demeanor lighter than usual, a stride more purposeful. I asked if she wanted to take a stroll with Kuma and me, and her reply was an enthusiastic *yes*. "I heard that," said the nurse.

The canteen wasn't open yet, so we traipsed around the "campus," which was how everyone referred to the hospital grounds. We passed billowing steam coming from the old Extended Care I and II units and arrived at the greenhouse, where Jill spent some of her time in a day program. Through the windows, I saw potted plants lined up on tables. Flowers and greenery were all thriving from the patients' care. Jill kept walking and didn't seem to notice.

I climbed the steps of the abandoned administration building, still boasting a historical marker, its significance belied by wood planks covering the second-story windows. Jill waited for me at the bottom of the stairs.

We circled the canteen three times, until the doors opened at noon. I offered Jill money, but she showed me she had her own and went inside. While I waited at one of the stone tables, an elderly woman shed her raincoat and fussed over my pretty dog. Hope was tinged with shame, as I found myself thinking how competent the woman was, wishing Jill could do as well when she was old.

The woman unwrapped a sandwich and offered a piece of crust to the dog. Then she moved to a table at the other end of the terrace.

Before I left the hospital that day, Jill and I sat side by side in the visitors' room, and I read Catherine's letter aloud. It was full of intimacies, as were all her missives. Knowing it would disappear if I left it with Jill, I tucked the letter back into my pocket. The documenter in me wanted to hold on to evidence of the relationship Catherine tried to maintain—this time, from a train on her way to New York City:

> *There are lakes and ponds I've been passing, with ducks, geese, and two white swans. They have lifted my spirits, which for no apparent reason dipped low last night and stayed that way this morning.*

Jill didn't respond to the letter, but she didn't appear to shut down. A young man wandered in, and from a corner, he slurred something I couldn't make out. All I heard was "show it to her." Thinking he was referring to the letter, I told him I'd already shown it to Jill. Then I realized he had unzipped his trousers and was about to loose his penis from white underpants.

Clutching Jill's hand, I led her briskly to the nurse's station and told the attendant what had happened. He looked exasperated. The young man ended up in the unit's "Education Corner" again. Jill grinned and seemed exhilarated by the commotion.

With an emphasis as strong as her earlier *yes*, she tugged on my arm, pulling me to the doorway of the men's area, adjacent to her own. She peered inside, and I felt the chasm between her world and mine, no matter how many letters I read or stories I told her. Although Jill had been a victim of the young man's aggression, she now appeared to align herself more with him than me. I knew I couldn't bridge that gap through effort. I returned home, felled by exhaustion, my shoulders aching.

⟋

When my father was in his eighties and still active, I joined him for lunch on the patio of a local restaurant under a striped umbrella. "Shoo," we said to a greedy grackle.

The frame of his glasses cut across his eyelids, his face familiar this way, but thinner recently. "I don't have the energy I did six months ago," he said.

Sometimes, he'd forget to call the hospital to see if Jill could come home. Sometimes, he didn't notice when she left her glasses behind. But he was there. He didn't look away.

"I won't do as much for her as you have." I spoke loudly so he'd hear me.

"I don't expect you to," he said.

"Maybe I'll move someplace cooler, far from hospitals."

"I gave up hoping at every turn," he said. "Now, I try to keep her safe. You'll do what you can, that's all."

But I was thinking: *Dad, I want to do much less than that.*

He stopped eating. After a minute, he asked if I'd noticed the girl with short blonde hair, overalls, and a tank top who was sitting near us on the patio—the girl with an elaborate, multicolored tattoo circling her smooth right armpit. My father smiled.

"Isn't that something?" he said, as we watched her reach her arms up and stretch.

PAIGE

~~~~~

DREW CICCOLO

Saturday, May 14, 2011

Woke early to attend Sarah's Brazilian jiu-jitsu tournament. Dad, sitting out back next to garden with legs crossed, said you were missing, or acting strangely, or a combination of both. Remarked that you hurried past him laughing when he saw you the night before, ran up the stairs laughing when he asked you how you were doing. Thought that was odd. I guess relapses are usually odd. Where was I the night before? Don't remember. Anyway, left house for jiu-jitsu tournament. Left Dad in the backyard.

First text I sent you, walking down sidewalk, 9:02 a.m.: *Dad had to go off his blood thinners to get infected teeth extracted on Monday . . . So he doesn't need to deal with any bullshit.*

Foolish of me to use the word "bullshit." Words have different implications for different people. To me, "bullshit" is nothing. To you, I can't be sure. Probably something. Probably not nothing. But I'd bitten my tongue so many times. I was just worried about the blood thinners. I still worry about Dad.

In any event, arrived at bus stop. Decided to skip Brazilian jiu-jitsu tournament. No need to go to ex-girlfriend's Brazilian jiu-jitsu tournament. Sort of pain in the ass, anyway. Hike to city and all. Decamp bus. Crowded Port Authority. Too many eyes trolling for weakness. Sarah's really into this Brazilian jiu-jitsu now. She posts pictures of herself on Facebook with bruises and black eyes from her training and her fights. Kind of bizarre. Violent. Seems to be on some sort of mission. Glad I'm not there to witness. Left bus stop and went about stupid day, which involved Starbucks and maybe Raymond's to eat and some amount of lying on Dan's couch.

Your response, 2:42 p.m.: *Drew I love u and always will but what a shitty text to get first thing in the am.*

Called you at 6:28 p.m., 6:43 p.m., 6:56 p.m.

Why didn't I call you until 6:28 p.m.? I was worried about you all day. That's the main reason I skipped the Brazilian jiu-jitsu tournament. I called people asking if they'd seen you. I called Jen. I called Brad. I called Kim. Did I call Lena? Spoke to Dad multiple times. He didn't know where you were.

Second text I sent you, 7:18 p.m.: *Where are you?*

Called you at 8:05 p.m.

Saw Scott outside of St. John's that night around 8:30 p.m. You were big fan of Scott. Conveyed my worry to Scott. He offered to drive me over to the house to check on you. Declined offer. Didn't think you were at house. Every time I spoke to Dad, he said you weren't home.

Called you at 8:42 p.m.

Instead of checking on you, went over to Dan's and watched movie on his couch, even though I'd been on same couch earlier in day. Thought you were at a bar or something. Thought relapse entailed only drinking. Pictured you sitting at bar getting hit on by "creepsters." Stupid.

Third text I sent you, 9:27 p.m.: *Are you ok?*

Called you at 10:13 p.m.

Got to house around midnight. Dad asked me to look in on you, to see if you were home yet.

Your light was on, the light by the door. Did I turn it on? Was it on already? From the doorway, it looked like you were sleeping. I almost didn't bother to call your name. I looked in through the doorway. It was a relief to see you in bed. Thought it good that you were home. I thought you were sleeping. I turned to walk across the hall. Did I turn to walk across the hall? I thought you were sleeping. I looked through the doorway. I called your name. You didn't move. I called your name. I thought you were sleeping. I called your name, maybe more delicately. I don't remember. I always liked saying your name. Your name is a good name. Some people's names aren't so easy to say. I called your name as I walked across the room. I called your name, and I touched you. I touched your leg first. I shook your leg. It didn't feel right. Then I touched your arm. I climbed onto the bed. Total attention and complete silence. I thought you were sleeping. The deep-red linen. Really, it was purple. Or maybe scarlet. The scarlet bed sheets. I can still see your face. Your mouth was open slightly, like you were sleeping. Your lips weren't the right color, too dark. A line of darkness at the bottom of your lip. I yelled your name. Your arm was cold. Your skin was your skin, but the color was different. There were dark colors in streaks on your shoulder and on your arm. I can still feel your body. I can still feel your leg and your arm. I can still see your arm and your shoulder. Your face is engraved in my mind. The phone curled in your hand. I can still see the blood welling under your skin. I can still feel exactly the way your skin felt. You were cold, but not freezing. I yelled your name. You had your phone in your hand. You weren't breathing. There were colors under your skin. I yelled your name. I grabbed you. I felt you. I remember your expression. You looked like yourself, but not like yourself.

I called 911. You still looked like yourself. My sister's not breathing. Help me. You were still. You weren't breathing. I called your name. Help me. Please. Help me. Put her flat on her back on a solid surface. I moved you. You were rigid. I moved you all the way off the bed. I was not me. You were not you. I was an instrument, a force to revive you. There must have been things on the bed. Your arms didn't move. Your arm stayed the same, except the phone had fallen by the bed. Your eyes moved, but not the right way. What was on the bed? Scarlet sheet. Scarlet pillowcase. Almost purple, the linen. Probably purple is the better word. I listened to the man on the phone. I checked for breath.

I did the compressions. A horrible sound came out of you. An empty sound. Your arms were fixed. I can still feel your body. I can still hear the sound that came from you. I breathed into your mouth. I can still taste your breath. I did everything perfectly. You were rigid. You were still. Your eyes were glass, different from your normal eyes. Your eyes were looking in the wrong direction, up and to the right. You were doll-like. I yelled your name. Your breath was the same as it was when we were little children. You had pure breath. I did the compressions. Why did that sound have to happen? I can still hear the sound. I can still feel your skin. I can still taste your breath. Your breath was the same as when we were little.

I made you cry in Southboro when I hit you with the lightsaber from *Star Wars*. I knew then—my sister is a girl, I can't hit her with the lightsaber. I'd never made you cry before. You were my sister. I called your name and I breathed into your mouth and I did the compressions. I heard Dad downstairs moaning. I can still hear him moaning. I couldn't control the volume of my voice. Things had to be controlled, so as not to upset. I messed up like when I hit you with the lightsaber. I didn't realize you were a girl and you didn't want to be hit with the lightsaber. Did I realize that? Was it some sort of test? Even if you were a boy, maybe the lightsaber would have made you cry. I cried because the hallway of the movie theater was so enormous. Then we got the lightsabers and I thought I was playing with you and you cried. I remember you crying. I remember your face at three years old. Were you two? Could you have been two? Was I four? Was

I five? No one has a face like that. No one has a face like your face. I did the compressions.

A police officer came in the bedroom door. I could hear Dad moaning downstairs. I heard him crying. The blood thinners. I heard more police boots on the stairs, police radios. He didn't know where you were. He didn't know you were home. He thought you were gone. The police got there before the paramedics. The police officer was young looking. I got the feeling he was a good person. He must have been younger than me. I can still feel the swirling inside my chest. Because of the adrenaline, I did everything perfectly. I did everything right. The police officer said you were in rigor mortis. He looked at me with humanity. She's been gone for hours. He was so young. That's why your arm was like that. Rigor mortis. I didn't know about any of that. I called your name and I felt your skin and they let me hold you. I didn't want them there. It was different from when I held Mom. The room was so messy. The room is still messy. Dad's house is always so messy. I put my face next to your face and held you. Your breath smelled pure, like a child's. I thought you were sleeping. I could hear him moaning downstairs. I could hear him crying. I went down. I left you. There were dark colors under your skin by your shoulder. I went down the stairs. I could hear him crying.

He looked up at me. What did he say? I don't want to remember what he said. There were police. He looked up at me. I sat next to him. I put my arm around him. I held his shoulder. He lowered his head. The blood thinners. His head was in his hands. I told him, we'll get through this. Words are sometimes useless. I told him, we'll find a way to get through this. He wanted his daughter. He didn't want me. I told him, we're going to get through this. I told him. He was making noises. The blood thinners. I told him, we will get through this. The police radios were in the house. Police radios are otherworldly in a house. Police radios never seem to sound right. I sat next to him. I told him. Then I moved around. I kept looking at things. The faded blue chair. The radiator.

I went back to your bedroom. You weren't breathing. I answered the questions. Alcohol. Drugs. Addict. Heroin. Hepatitis-C. You were on the floor. I held you on the floor. I put my cheek against your cheek. Your mouth was open. You had perfect teeth. My teeth are ugly. You had lovely white teeth. There were marks on your shoulder and your arm. That's where the blood went. You weren't breathing. You were still. Why did I leave the room? The medical examiner. What was said? The sounds that came out of me were horrible. There were a lot of bad sounds that night. I couldn't control them. I've never cried like that. You were home the whole time.

Humans have been on the earth for about 200,000 years. We still don't know what to do. 200,000 years is not enough time. The person must stay in the house. The person must stay in the house for a period of time. You have to hold the person. I understood that when Mom died. The person needs to stay in the house for longer than they let them. The person needs to be held. The person needs to be kissed. The tears must go into their skin. This is not grotesque. The person needs to stay for a period of time. This is not the custom here. Your eyes were looking in the wrong direction, up and to the right. Mom's eyes were closed.

I moved Dad into the kitchen before they carried you out the door. They left their plastic gloves in your bedroom.

I called Dan. He was the first to come. I remember his face, too. Then the rest: Sanjay, Kim, Jen, Brad. Sanjay stayed all night and into the morning on the couch downstairs. It rained for a week straight. It really did. Every day. I didn't eat. Then I started by eating a banana. Then another banana. A bottle of water here. A banana there.

You were home the whole time. I take good care of Frankie. She gets only the most expensive cat food. She is very pampered. She sleeps with me every night. Usually, she insists on getting under the covers and curling up. You were home the whole time. I started drinking 5hr Energies soon after you died because I felt like I couldn't focus and couldn't write. I still drink them. I'm hooked. It's horrible. Some girl told me I'm going to get eyebrow cancer. You would laugh about it maybe. You were home the whole time. Remember when we hadn't seen each other for a long time and you came downstairs and I was sitting at the dining-room table? You said I looked like Jim Morrison, then paused and said: on his way down. I always remember that. It was good comedic timing. Scott offered to drive me to check on you. You were funny and smarter than me and always had it more together. You were home the whole time. The therapist prescribed me Vistaril, a non-narcotic anxiety medication in case

I had panic attacks. The therapist said I had to talk about finding you, so as not to get PTSD. Scott offered to drive me. You were home the whole time.

Elephants. Grief, and maybe even regret, aren't specific to humans. Elephants grieve for extended periods of time. Elephants hold vigils for their dead, especially if it's a dead child. They try to revive them. They look slumped and sad. Elephants have died of grief. They have special camps for elephants whose families have been killed. They have to become attached to the humans, or they'll die of grief. This is my take, anyway. It's piecemeal. Documentary, Internet, etc. Maybe from a documentary I saw at Dan's house. Who the fuck knows. Elephants.

In your bedroom, I found a tall boot filled with vodka bottles. Your breath is still inside of me. I have all of the stuff you wrote while you were home, and all the letters you sent me when you were away. I haven't been able to read any of them, because I know what will happen. Or because I don't know what will happen. I also can't look at pictures of you. Your breath is still inside of me. You were home the whole time. And where was I? And why couldn't I protect you? Why couldn't I ever seem to protect you? I thought you were sleeping. And you were home the whole time. I can still taste your breath.

Your funeral was the most crowded funeral I've ever seen, not that I've seen so many funerals or anything. I paid for the floral arrangement. I think you would have liked it. Michelle spoke. Lena spoke. I spoke. Dad spoke. Mrs. Myers spoke. This is the poem I picked for your prayer card:

Do not stand at my grave and weep:
I am not there, I do not sleep.
I am a thousand winds that blow:
I am the diamond glints on snow.
I am the sunlight on ripened grain:
I am the gentle autumn rain.
When you awaken in the
morning's hush,
I am the swift uplifting rush
of quiet birds in circled flight.
I am the soft star that shines at night.
Do not stand at my grave and cry.
I am not there: I did not die.

I don't even know what it means. I mean, I do, but I don't. I still sit on Dan's couch. We found a British television show called *Peep Show,* which I think you'd get a kick out of. Sometimes when I'm walking around, I want to rip my chest open and release myself to the universe.

I'd like to do something special with your ashes. Dad wants his and Mom's spread in the ocean near Falmouth on Cape Cod. I think I will take you lots of places with me and spread you where I think you'd like to be, far away from deep-red linen, scarlet bed sheets, lightsabers, walkie talkies, Brazilian jiu-jitsu tournaments, radiators, and faded blue chairs.

Source

"Do Not Stand at My Grave and Weep" by Mary Elizabeth Frye. Frye wrote the poem in 1932 and never published it, although she made a number of copies for friends.

ARRIVAL

Writing gives voice to the chaos and the beauty and the passion and the grief. It helps me to experience the world more deeply and to process what the universe chooses to throw in my direction. It's a joy so pure that when I'm unable to do it, I feel as if one of my hands has been lopped off, an eye plucked out.

—Kim Triedman

CLIMBING THE WALLS

JOANNA BRICHETTO

Four years ago, I started a garden project—a trellis—hoping for a wall of vines I'd be able to admire from the kitchen. It took time to work out details, rummage for supplies, realize cypress would need a pilot hole for each screw, scoot the ladder across the porch eaves without puncturing the screen wall. I'd also need a stone-lined bed to give vines root room.

The surprise was that I had the strength to do any of this: to haul limestone, gouge bindweed, slap the hammer, even to just keep climbing the lopsided ladder. Usually, I would have gotten a migraine or pulled a muscle or become so disgusted at the snowballing complications of each step I would have abandoned the project as yet another undoable DIY. But I didn't. I started. I finished.

The stamina and positivity were new. They were new *pills*. One drug gave me energy. Another drug slowed my central nervous system enough to suppress chronic migraines—I get at least three a week—and to relax the hyper-vigilant, hyper-crippling inner voice. I felt great. I couldn't keep still or stop my legs from trying to walk, twitch, and tap, but I felt *great*. I could hang a trellis all by myself no matter how long it took and I didn't get tired or even have to stop and eat.

I talked faster. Way faster. I talked like I hammered those nails, with quick, easy swings, but from a crooked place. If you lean your ladder against screen, you fall.

When I walked through doorways, I'd reach up to slap the lintel, like boys do when they're suddenly tall enough. I didn't need food; I needed to walk and walk and walk and do. I wasn't afraid to make phone calls, I didn't procrastinate returning merchandise to stores, I grocery shopped without panic, I volunteered as a visiting naturalist at my son's preschool. I kept moving, moving forward, not just reacting to things but making the world react to *me*. I was making the ripples, not just negotiating waves.

My sister said she liked it. My clothes fit better, and then I had to get new ones that were smaller.

The doctor who gave me these pills assessed me quickly. He prescribed and turned me over to a nurse. My appointments with her were brief "med checks"—industry standard at ten minutes, tops. I reported my symptoms; she tweaked my drugs. I barely slept. Nurse added a drug for that. Soon, I was on four drugs. And when I started breaking through the screen—not just stretching, but breaking through the membrane between sane and not sane, alive and wanting not to be, she added another. And that's when I fell.

I don't want to remember this. Four years isn't long. Recovering from what I'm afraid to describe took a full year.

~~

Coming back, I looked anorexic. I couldn't sleep. I wanted to die, and I thought of ways I might die without suicide negating the life-insurance benefits my husband would need for child care. I had a constant tremor; my body vibrated like a tuning fork without the tune. I was a ghost looking at my family. I watched them busy without me. I could see them, but I made no impact, no mark. I floated in spinning confusion and loss, and I had no rest, no rest, not one moment of peace.

There were utility blades in the toolbox. There were pills, of course, left over. The only gun was a Red Ryder BB in the attic. There was the car, but I could barely shuffle across a room, much less drive. I asked to go with the family to school drop-off every morning. I wanted to see my boy and girl walk hand-in-hand toward the building. This was what I'd envisioned when the little one was born: that my kids would be a kindergartener and a high school senior the same year at the same school, and I needed to see it, to be there, *to not be dead*, and if I saw it, I might be able to remember it later and feel not just the grasping pain but the happiness, too, like taking a photograph with the hope that you'll appreciate it later.

I did take a photograph. I did appreciate it later. I still do.

But to keep my brain from swirling like a full toilet right when it's about to overflow—when the mass rises instead of falls, and there is no plunger or cut-off valve, and it's not your house, and there is carpet, and there are things in the toilet from both ends of your body, and it's the middle of the night—to keep my brain from spinning out of my scalp, I had to anchor it to something else that moved, too, like to the trees outside the car window. The trees didn't move, obviously, but I moved past them in the passenger seat. I named them, *identified* them, which meant I had to remember species from far back in the fog, but luckily, there were a lot of hackberries, because Nashville is the hackberry capital of the world, even though no one but me knows this or cares, and I concentrated as best I could, brought my mind to bear as I aimed at each one: hackberry, elm, hackberry, dogwood, Osage orange, sugar maple, hackberry, hackberry.

I thanked them. Thank you, hackberry. Thank you, walnut. Thank you, sweetgum. Thank you, willow oak. Thanking them saved me.

Years before, when I was just normal crazy—Depression and Generalized Anxiety—I went to a school lecture about anxious teens because my teen was anxious (big surprise), and the expert said that anxiety and gratitude were mutually exclusive. He said a gratitude journal could work wonders, could reframe all, could ease the balance back toward calm. He was calm. He said that if you were anxious, then you were not grateful enough. *If, then.* Which made me more anxious, because obviously I deserved to be anxious if I couldn't whip gratitude up to therapeutic levels.

It took years for me to realize he was full of shit. Not that gratitude doesn't help, because it does, but because gratitude and anxiety are not mutually exclusive and in fact can interlock the holy hell out of each other, can grip the same moment in time, the same breath, the same pulse in my skin so pale that I can see the blue and red under it, see where to aim a utility blade. Gratitude and terror. Two sides of the coin, two edges of the sword, Janus-faced, pick a metaphor for the reality that they are *mutually inclusive.*

The same expert still gives the lecture with the same title at the same school to new waves of parents, but I am done with him.

I still can't write about the crescendo and climax of crazy, but I will say it happened at the beach, on vacation. And because I telephoned the nurse twice during that week so I could ask if what I was experiencing was normal, the doctor fired me. Cut me off. Said I needed more help than their office was prepared to give. I heard this via the nurse on that second call. Perhaps an inpatient facility would be more my cup of tea. They drugged me; they fired me. *If, then.*

On my own medical advice, I stopped all meds cold turkey 600 miles from home. That's when the screen broke, and I broke. If there were visible scars from such a thing, my skin would be as ridged and scabbed as hackberry bark. Hackberry bark is easily identifiable from a moving car at any speed.

When I was finally brought back home, everything seemed oddly familiar. I used to live here. Birdseed. I used to feed birds.

Art supplies. I used to teach children. These things were my things. I had forgotten. My things reminded me I had once been a real person.

They were not enough.

My mom came for a visit to feed me, as good moms do, but mine is a registered nurse, which was a bonus. She brought a recliner, because I couldn't lie flat. I watched her haul it out of her van, the footrest kicking forward to knock her off-balance, and a yard guy next door ran over to help. She set it up in the bedroom with blankets, because I could never get warm. Good friends came by and brought treats I couldn't yet taste.

Lamaze breathing helped. Lamaze is old-school and not often taught at birthing classes now, but it saved me with both labors when my babies took forever to come out, and the epidurals didn't work, and both transition phases took me straight to hell, and all I could do was stare at the fingers my husband held up that told me how many times to breathe: *hee, hee, hee, hoo*. It looks like laughter when I type it, and Lamaze is easy to ridicule, but it's real. It's the regulation of breath, the living breath. It can get you to the next revolution of a second hand on a clock, which is sometimes all you have.

Upon reflection, I have to amend my toilet analogy. It is fairly accurate for the beginning swirls, but not for the middle, which I'm leaving out. With a toilet, the volume of liquid underneath the filth is finite: an American Standard tankful of city water only, no more. But the volume of whatever was rising in me was the ocean, limitless, unknown, a hurricane, the Bering Sea in those terrifying YouTube videos. And all I could do was react to the waves around me. Tread water like the counselors taught at Girl Scout camp. Tread water and keep breathing, make those patterns with my breath.

Two more things helped. I made marks. This is legit art jargon: We make marks with tools. A soft-lead pencil and a pad of paper proved I existed, because I could make marks with them. I doodled tessellations, which again looks kind of funny to type here—*doodle*—but I made semi-circles that connected to each other: newest to next newest, segments of one long caterpillar that snaked across the drawing paper. There was no discrete shape; they were all linked together. Nothing floated alone.

The other thing was a person. My husband made me look in his eyes, made me see myself reflected in his irises, to see proof that I was there. We did this a lot during the time I can't describe. It made the noise crank down a level, from *Spinal Tap* eleven to ten. And he reminded me every day, every night, that he loved me and needed me and the kids loved me and needed me, and I wrote this over and over and over in the cream-colored sketch pad opposite the pages of caterpillar tessellations, and when I wasn't writing these words, I read them, carried them under my fattening arm. They were my mantra.

In the car, I still identified trees.

The swirls did slow, the fog cleared, the ground returned. I don't understand the physiology of what happened and why it took so long to recover after I stopped the drugs, why the collateral damage outlasted published pharmaceutical half-lives and gave me less than half a life. Drug-induced supersensitivity psychosis is my best guess, but to investigate further would trigger too much anxiety. I never did complain to or about the doctor, and I am terrified I'll have to take another drug for something someday and that my husband will not be there to pull me back and I will fall through and stay.

> To suffer is not redemption.
> *We are not redeemed by suffering.*
> To suffer is to suffer.
> Whether a scratch or a psyche, the wound is what we are.

There is no new doctor; there are no drugs. Anxiety and gratitude continue to rub along on opposites sides of a thin coin, but I cultivate the latter as often as I can, which is often. I am with my family. I learn new trees. Every day I make marks of some kind on some thing in some way. I am here.

Meanwhile, my trellis looks ready to guide another summer of morning glories straight up to the sky.

LOOSE ASSOCIATIONS

~

CARL BOWLBY

Loose Association #1

It's ironic to realize my psychotherapist is finished with me. Sarah says she's leaving her Massachusetts employer, CSO (Clinical and Support Options), to be near two of her children and a grandchild on the West Coast. She says she's sorry, she needs to reschedule our appointment, and how am I feeling about that? Abandoned. But.

Apparently, Sarah (not her real name) is going to open up her own private practice there. She says "West Coast," but I know through our myriad conversations over the past decade she's going to Portland, Oregon—a place I've never been, but have heard plenty about. You know, the millennials of Portland: tattooed, pierced, arty, hip, coffee-addicted. Brewers of the self-proclaimed microbrew capital of the US. Contrary to whatever anybody tells you about the Pacific Northwest, though, it rains—a lot! Ever hear of suicide capital Seattle, Washington?

From what I know of Sarah, she's a copper penny in a dime store. She's just not going to fit in. She's never revealed her age to me, but my best guess is 68, even 70. What is she going to do in a location consisting mainly of hipsters? Will Sarah get a tattoo out there? Pierce her septum? Get a belly ring? Dye her hair purple? Well, in reality, she has already dyed her hair blonde with a streak or two of purple. So, maybe she *is* prepping herself for the onslaught of techy twenty-somethings.

And I might as well tell you now, before I truly lose my train of thought, that the very reason I've been seeing Sarah all these years is because of a referral from her daughter, Bette (none of these names are real), whom I met around 2003, when she was living briefly in the Berkshires. So, Bette was really my first step on the path leading into the therapy world. Bette—it should be obvious by now—is one of the daughters who has relocated to Portland. I like to think I know Bette pretty well. Well enough to label her with the sexist moniker "Big Boobs Bette."

Loose Association #2

I'm with Sarah because I have schizoaffective disorder, a diagnosis handed down to me by a young psychiatrist in Berlin, Vermont, about a year before Bette. It's why I collect Social Security disability pay. The mother of my child (our child) has something like what I have. Except worse. She is the mother of loose associations. Take Berlin. Berlin, Germany? Well, maybe, if you were to listen in on our disconnected and rambling conversations. And we have a child together, a beautiful, Berlin-born girl who is now sixteen. She gives me a reason to live. And I have her to myself, because her mother handed her over to me in a parking garage in Montpelier, Vermont.

Loose Association #3

I don't live in Montpelier now. My daughter and I are in the Berkshires of western Massachusetts, and, if you've ever been here, you know what I'm talking about.

You may have heard of Tanglewood, where the Boston Symphony Orchestra has played every summer since the 1930s. The "Shed" was christened the "Serge Koussevitzky Music Shed" in the 1980s after the BSO conductor who first played there. Wikipedia says Tanglewood takes its name from the nineteenth-century American author Nathaniel Hawthorne's short-story collection *Tanglewood Tales,* which was published in 1853 after he had left his little red farmhouse in Lenox, Massachusetts—his brief stint in the Berkshires, which he did not like when all is said and done.

Loose Association #4

So, while I may be *graduating* from what I often refer to as "therapy class" with Sarah, she's leaving *me* after ten years of intense psychoanalysis and energy work, in which she attempted to unravel my psychic distress, with varying degrees of success, from growing up with a family of cruel narcissists.

Add to the mix an older brother who liked to use me for his *frottage* indulgences. It's a French word. I'm part French-Canadian.

He pretended many years later, when I angrily confronted him about his sexual assaults (at the suggestion of Sarah), that what he did had absolutely *no* effect on my developing brain as a small child. I mean, Christ, I was what, five years old? Six? At any rate, I was very young when this fifteen-year-old predator rubbed himself against me.

A lot of us mentally ill types have had an "originating trauma" of sexual abuse that mirrors our disabled mental capacities later into young adulthood and beyond. Some might call these "triggers" or "crisis moments." And then there are the drugs.

Disordered Thought #1

And then there's Dr. M.

I have a medical doctor who's treating my substance-abuse condition, which he calls a disease of the brain. He's already suggested I read two books on the topic. The first book gets into the costly drug war and promotes across-the-board legalization. The second book, which I haven't finished yet, gets into the medical and technical details of why a childhood filled with sexual assaults often results in adult substance abuse.

Disordered Thought #2

Sarah annoys me when she pries into my experiences with Dr. M. Truthfully, I think it's none of her damn business. I just think she's a gossip. I tell her that everything is going fine, and I'm doing fine, and no, no, I'm not using drugs. Which is a lie. I might as well tell you now that my idea of psychotherapy isn't to reveal everything that goes on in my life. Maybe it's a self-defensive gesture, but there are certain things I don't go public with. With anyone. Not even with my precious Sarah.

Disordered Thought #3

I like listening to classic jazz. I'm pitifully tired of making *sense*. I long to let it all out, everything, in one wild, stormy tangent and be done with it. You know, kind of like Jack Kerouac. Nobody cares, anyway, except self-absorbed people who are obsessed with labeling things, putting me in a box like a corpse stuffed in its coffin.

Sarah is never my grim reaper, however. She never puts me in a box. She welcomes all facets of my troubled *mood disorder*. "All is welcome here," she often says during our sessions.

Disordered Thought #4

All is welcome here, indeed—except for being on time. Oh, how it grates on my nerves when Sarah leaves me in the sad waiting room at CSO, as she did just yesterday. I bring my e-reader with me to stifle the boredom, but Sarah is so often late it's become a "thing" with us. She says "sorry" again (and again), and I give her a smirk, implying I'm not pleased, and then we saunter down the corridor to her office, where she makes her excuse. This time she had to "send a document."

Really? You had to keep me waiting, which you know I loathe, just so you could send a document that could have been sent before our appointed time? I don't get it. It's as if she's being rebellious to test my reaction. And while my inner demon wants to lash out, I restrain myself. I turn into the polite self that Sarah's been trying to nurture in me since we began seeing one another.

Disordered Thought #5

As I've said, I'm tired of making sense. Disordered thoughts and loose associations are inbred. Schizotypal personality disorder, as I've heard it's now called—or SAD for schizoaffective disorder, to initialize the thing, though it's not to be confused with seasonal affective disorder. SAD 1 and SAD 2. I have SAD 1. But don't tell that to my "pill lady" (my nurse practitioner, Carol, who gives me meds for what she insists is only bipolar disorder—it, too, was a popular diagnosis at one time).

I may be manic sometimes, but I'm not bipolar. I have many conversations out loud with myself precisely concerning this ongoing disagreement. With myself.

Carol has also been irritating me lately. We had a session recently where she ignited my panic. Because Sarah was leaving CSO, Carol had to "close my case." What? She then said she "has a private practice" and can see me in my home. My first reaction was *not in my house!* But I played along (as I usually do) and said that would be fine, all the while stifling the adrenaline-rush of panic. Sometimes, I think CSO makes me crazy. Maybe it's all their fault. But this could only be "magical thinking" or "delusional."

You pick.

Disordered Thought #6

I call SAD 1 cases "schizophrenic-lite." Those of us who are on the edge of full-blown hallucinatory existences have to put up with voices just the same. We can hear and identify the voices in our head, but don't literally hear them speaking out loud.

I also obsess over things to a shocking degree. I'm a checker. Check the wallet. Check the keys. Lock the doors. Close the windows. Make sure my meds are in my lunch bag, which I take with me everywhere. Don't step on cracks. Drive in the middle of my car lane. Without meds, I might as well be schizophrenic.

Loose Association #5

People come, and people go, and so it is with my Sarah. Bye-bye. Go off to Portland and be with the millennial hipsters who are generationally underfed—or is it overfed? No matter. Young and clever, most of them. Wannabes or pretentious. I'm too singular to be pretentious. To be truly pretentious, you have to belong to a group or be connected with some movement that makes you part of a group.

"Just breathe," I can hear Sarah softly telling me.

Sorry, Sarah. Breathing deeply, consciously, can't cure mental illness.

Loose Association #6

Those of you reading this who aren't supported by family and government for your daily bread are typically functional humans. The rest of us *dys*functional types need assistance to get through life. That's really the only difference between you and me. I hear the voices inside other people saying, "I hope [he, she, it] gets the help [he, she, it] needs." I hate that. I *am* getting help. I'm on meds. I get a government paycheck for being thoroughly unemployable.

Loose Association #7

It's tough to be Generation X. We were done before we even began.

Now I'm thinking of my deceased sister-in-law. She died at the age of 46 of cancer in October 2015. She was a beacon in a world of calumny and bitterness. She was bright, alive, and spar-kling—*and* she didn't smoke or drink booze. Clean as a whistle. But the cancer was all over her body.

On Memorial Day the following year, in a tribute to her battle with cancer, my sister from Queens planted a tree. Good for her. I didn't attend the ceremony for various reasons. My brother—my sister-in-law's husband—had already gotten on with his "new life" without her: a new car; a trip to San Diego, to Puerto Rico; a new girlfriend ordering furniture for a new house.

When I think of Sarah leaving me for Portland, I see a candle snuffing out in the darkened room of my psyche, a lighthouse going dark before my storm-tossed ship—and a whole host of other metaphors.

Epilogue 2016

A month ago, Sarah suddenly informed me, via iMessage, that she's calling off her move indefinitely.

"Really?" I asked (and pinched) myself repeatedly. "Are you sure?"

She said yes, she's staying put. I am thrilled beyond words. All the worry, my sense of loss and panic, has lifted, *deus-ex-machina* style. Simply put, there are certain irreplaceable people who make living bearable.

The End (indefinitely)

PLUCKING AND PREENING

LINDA SASLOW

The summer when I was eight, I started pulling out my own hair, strand by strand. In 1978, my parents were newly divorced with joint custody, which meant I made a twice-monthly, ninety-minute trek from California's San Gabriel Valley to San Clemente in the back seat of my mother's tan Pontiac Firebird. Most kids would have been thrilled to head to a beach town like San Clemente for the weekend. Instead, I sat quietly, pulling strawberry-blonde hairs from the top of my scalp while Neil Diamond played on the eight-track tape deck, the back seat littered with cast-off curls.

When I was nine or so, my mother's hairdresser friend who cut my hair commented on a little bald spot at the top of my head and the fountain of short re-grown hairs. I know my mother knew about the hair plucking, but she never took me to any sort of therapy. She may have scolded me for the behavior, but it wasn't effective.

Most of my life, I assumed—wrongly informed as I'd been by non-professionals—that this condition was related to self-mutilation. It's not. But several other impulse-control disorders are: promiscuity, kleptomania, fire starting, and various daily fixations. I've been happily married for more than two decades, so the first condition has its own balm. Those second and third buggy brain farts have never been an issue.

But daily fixations? Compulsive gambling is a kissing cousin to compulsive hair pulling. While I loathe Las Vegas-style gambling, flipping a coin up to ten times a day is the norm for me. Other everyday decisions I determine with a coin flip: where I'm going to eat my tuna poke lunch bowl, where to drink my soy mocha, whether or not to attend a Saturday kundalini yoga class. My iPhone has a coin-flipping app in case a real penny isn't handy.

My grandmother's death led to a few weeks of compulsive tugging when I was nearly forty years old. Recently, my husband hiked Peru's Inca Trail to Machu Picchu and was away from cell phone towers for four days. I pulled my hair in a frenzy then. My bipolar meds were inadequate. I drank quite a bit, which felt bad for other reasons.

I'm also dogged by a related condition known as intermittent explosive disorder—displays of anger disproportionate to the situation at hand. In my late thirties, when my children spilled candy on the kitchen floor and tried to save it to eat later, I threw a giant box of See's Valentine's chocolates in the garbage despite their heated protests. At times, such anger has led to the balkanization of my own home, a thought that still saddens me.

The behavioral therapy "spotting" techniques of Recovery International, which I spent seven years espousing as a support

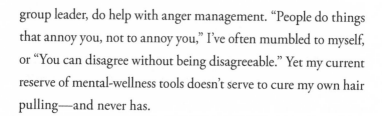

group leader, do help with anger management. "People do things that annoy you, not to annoy you," I've often mumbled to myself, or "You can disagree without being disagreeable." Yet my current reserve of mental-wellness tools doesn't serve to cure my own hair pulling—and never has.

Hair pulling disorder (HPD) is also known as trichotillomania. When I first heard the term *trichotillomania* from my primary care physician, I had to go to a psychologist to find out what it meant. I was almost forty when I first mentioned my condition to a therapist, and I've never seen anyone who specializes in treating HPD.

Experts disagree about whether anxiety is the true trigger, although some researchers have found a link to parental divorce and separation. The most recent edition of the *Diagnostic and Statistical Manual of Mental Disorders* (*DSM-5*) classifies trichotillomania in its chapter with obsessive-compulsive and related disorders. The *DSM-5* says the condition can be related to skin picking. Boredom can also cause people to pluck and preen.

I'll admit that popping a zit feels far more fun than it should, so maybe I have a touch of skin-picking disorder, too, but nothing that merits special treatment. I'm guilty of sitting on the couch in front of a nerve-racking television show like *Breaking Bad* while unconsciously my hands hit my scalp. I enjoy the tugging sensation of the hair being liberated from my skin. If the follicle is attached and can be stripped from the strand, it's even more pleasurable. If I were a network news junkie, I'd be absolutely bald.

The *DSM-5* estimates that up to 2 percent of the adult and adolescent population is afflicted with trichotillomania. A 2010 paper in *Clinical Psychology Review* estimated that three million individuals in the United States suffer from the disorder. Pinning down numbers for a condition like this, especially one that didn't even have a fancy name until recently, is tricky. But backed by a number of research studies and clinical observation, the *DSM-5* states that women are far more likely to pull their hair compulsively than men, at a ratio of 10:1.

Here's the truly crazy thing: I spend a minimum of $120 every six weeks to get my hair colored, highlighted, and cut to keep up with the Real Housewives of Orange County. From an HPD standpoint, I'm tossing aside expensive strands I could pull myself—that I want to pull badly. If I begin to suffer from age-related hair loss, as my 75-year-old mother does, this seemingly benign habit may morph into something that requires aggressive cognitive behavioral therapy, the preferred way to treat hair pulling when it becomes extreme.

Benzodiazepines and SSRIs can dull my urges, but they aren't one hundred percent effective. I pull my hair out less if I've been drinking, but this isn't a healthy solution, and after the Inca Trail binge, I'm now sober. At age 48, I've spent six months on Lithium, and the hair pulling is down to something I do involuntarily once a month. If I'm in a particularly plucky mood, I might put on a beret or arrange my hair in a topknot.

Fortunately, I'm never tempted to tear at the thin hair on my arms and legs.

I've taken a twice-daily cocktail of psychiatric medication for bipolar disorder since I was 28, a far more serious condition that flares up about every ten years. But my hair pulling has, without a whisper of doubt, worsened as I've aged. My therapist blames it on perimenopause, when the condition can actually take on an explosive life of its own, a slew of experts claim. What the experts don't say is that it's not just about hormones; at this stage of life, the residue of the world's cruelty toward women is just sinking in.

I'm lucky. My hair loss is barely detectable and doesn't mar my outward appearance. When I was in my mid-forties, my neuropsychologist told me she wouldn't consider treating me for HPD unless I was missing an eyebrow. Still, there are protracted phases of my life where I've routinely pulled out at least three hairs from somewhere on my body every day.

I usually attack my scalp and pubic region. The coarser and thicker the hair, the better it is to harvest and the more victorious I feel. Once, I cashed in a coupon for a free bikini wax, but in the end felt cheated that I couldn't enjoy yanking the hairs myself. And the woman spreading the Popsicle stick of hot black goop on my privates seemed excessively aloof. Maybe there isn't a lot of fun in pulling out another person's hair, especially if it's just a job.

(Spoiler alert for those wishing to save money at the salon: My hair-removal method sometimes causes unsightly ingrown hairs that mar my pale Irish skin for months. I also don't wear mascara because it thickens the consistency of my red lashes, drawing my hands to them. The solution is to have them professionally dyed dark brown every couple of months.)

The *DSM-5* notes that some hair pullers are conscious of the behavior and others aren't. For some, it's automatic; for others, it's a conscious activity. For me, when I pluck hairs on my head and in my nether region, it's unconscious at first. But once that thick and wiry strand is in my grasp, I'm fully aware. I love the feeling. I bask in the microburst of anxiety release. Plucking and preening can even produce a Zen-like state.

As I run my fingers down its stalk and over the root, my mind focuses on the hair's smoothness or coarseness, the color variation of the individual strand. I rarely pull more than three in succession. I'm nearly always alone and in a private space. The bathroom, the bed, and the car stalled behind the five-mile-an-hour freight train are perfect opportunities to indulge.

⟜

Now that I'm nearing menopause, I have stray hairs on my neck and chin. I go after these relentlessly each night with tweezers. While the *DSM-5* would characterize my grooming as "normative hair removal," pulling these stubby and wiry facial hairs is an intense rush. I doubt it excites the average person in this way, but unless I end up clawing my face apart,

I wouldn't consider electrolysis or facial waxing. It would eliminate the chase.

I set aside time before bed to tweeze a minimum of three hairs from my neck and chin while gazing in the bathroom mirror. Some people meticulously floss their teeth; I wind down at the end of my daily treadmill of English tutoring by picking the hairs on my chin and neck and eyebrows. Finding a gray eyebrow strand is a significant triumph. I like to collect each tiny hair in my left palm and run my fingers over the coarse strands before I discard them in the toilet.

It's my absolution; it's my reward. It's not painful. There's nothing but a quick tugging sensation. It's not masochistic. A few minutes of weeding my own body of hair that's defiant and aberrantly wiry is like a mental push of the button on the emotional morphine pump.

I used to be so ashamed. In college, if one of my dorm-mates asked about my fixation, I rebuffed her. I hid my neurosis. But in my early twenties, after I'd met the man who became my husband, one of his sisters admitted to me that she liked to "pick her curlies," too. We went on to share the challenges of our mutual madness, and this sisterhood has allowed me to become more open about the disorder.

"There sure are a lot of dusty tangles of red hair in our bedroom," my husband sometimes complains after he vacuums our house. "Is it spring shedding season?"

Like a loyal landscaper, thinning the thistles among the lilies, my toil will never cease.

Sources

Diagnostic and Statistical Manual of Mental Disorders (*DSM-5*), edited and published by the American Psychiatric Association, 2013 (and 2017 supplement).

"Trichotillomania: A Current Review" by D.C. Duke *et al.*, *Clinical Psychology Review,* 2010.

THE LONGEST WALK

KIM TRIEDMAN

My life broke right down the middle—cleanly, like a dried-out stick. There was no warning, no way any of us could have seen it coming. One moment, I was a young mother sitting on a Boston stoop, my three daughters shrieking and giggling through the open window behind me. The next, I was overcome by an anxiety so utterly airless and paralyzing that my throat sealed over. The midsummer sky seemed to go abruptly white, as if color itself had been called into question.

No one tells you how far away depression takes you. From your life. From your loved ones. From the only self you've ever known. From time as you've always experienced it. The insulation borders on incarceration—a cocoon made of threads so fine and gauzy and tenacious that only the tiniest flickers of light are allowed in or out. You do it alone. You go through it without company or consolation. It grabs you from behind, tears you from everything familiar and reasonable and dangles you, howling, over the precipice.

Today, after 22 long years of hindsight, I've come to think of depression as an inability to imagine the future—to extrapolate beyond the endless, borderless, terrifying present.

Your husband sits down next to you on the stoop and says, "Just *stop* it," as though you have any say in the matter.

Your sister says, "Get a haircut—you just need a little pampering," as though that has any meaning whatsoever.

Your mother says, "Please, *please,* just eat the sandwich," as though her heart is breaking.

⟳

My mother-in-law, who went through decades of disabling and wrenching health problems, was one of the most non-depressed people I've ever known. She made me realize that had someone else lived my life, he or she might have barreled through it unscathed. There was no bogeyman, no criminal neglect. I was blessed with loving parents and abundant emotional support. But throughout my childhood and early adulthood, I was also exquisitely sensitive, quick to well up, as if my skin were wafer-thin. I thrummed to the emotional tremors of those around me, prey to the vicissitudes of other people's internal weather.

But it was a life, and I lived it well. I worked and fell in love and bought a house and brought three amazing children into the world. It was a strong and sturdy thing, or so I believed. By my mid-thirties—as my last daughter approached preschool age—I felt I'd arrived at a midpoint, where most of life's big surprises were behind me and the future spilled out like something comfortable and known. Put another way, I assumed this was where my life began to end. I'd always know what room I would wake up in and what I'd see when I looked out my bedroom window. As time rolled on, I'd have more and more to look back on but less to dream about.

Then the sky went white. My brain hissed with the sound of a thousand coiled snakes. Life turned on its head, and for the first time, I had absolutely no idea what my future held.

A few long days later, with some hastily prescribed Xanax propping me up, I landed in a psychiatrist's office, terrified. He was middle-aged—tall and loose-limbed and remote—and as I shook his hand, I knew nothing would ever be the same.

It was as though I'd landed on a different planet, with an entirely different trajectory, an orbit that circled my old life but only from a distance. I'd had no direct experience with mental illness or therapy or psychoactive medications. I wasn't certain what was wrong with me, but I assumed the worst. Another thing no one tells you is that anxiety goes hand-in-glove with depression. When my psychiatrist broke this news, I wept with gratitude. At least I wasn't psychotic.

I saw him only a few times. The Prozac would take weeks to kick in, and I knew I was in no shape to take care of myself, let alone my daughters. My husband was running his own business and traveled extensively; he didn't have room to step into that role. So we decamped to my mom and dad's home in southern Rhode Island, the girls and I, and settled in for whatever came next.

For the six or so weeks that I was severely depressed, the overriding emotion I felt was fear. Nothing I'd known prepared me for how it breathes its own dark into you—the way it inhabits you as you inhabit it. Random things unhinged me: the evening news, a quality of light, the clots of dirty laundry metastasizing in the bedroom corners. I stared at a light switch on the wall one evening and felt the creep of black terror just behind my right shoulder.

I no longer knew how to take care of myself: I could scarcely eat or sleep or hold a conversation. I lost track of time. For weeks, I existed on dry Cheerios and ginger ale and coffee-flavored Ensure—the only foods I was able to abide, choked down under the watchful eye of my mother.

During that time, my kids were allowed into my room for only short visits with either my mother or father. I was aware of their hushed, careful, little-girl trepidation, their desperate efforts not to cry. But I knew I couldn't touch them, could neither take them in nor give myself to them. It was too painful to see in their eyes the questions and fears I knew I couldn't ease. In my memory of that time, they were just three faces—disembodied, oversized, and out of focus, floating in and out of the ether like malarial dreams.

So, too, with my friends, who either fell away or didn't know how to talk to me. None of my siblings had been through anything similar or could find a way to talk about it. I even felt a growing distance from my husband, whose brilliant sense of humor had won me over nearly twenty years earlier but now served only to remind me that he didn't fathom how thoroughly irrelevant humor was.

I knew he was scared. I knew he had to keep working. I knew that—like me—he had no tools for dealing with this new and alarming reality. But his attempts to jolly me out of my depression just made me feel more alone.

Only my mother seemed to know what to do. She knew how to *not* talk. After hours cowering in a dark room, hidden under my covers, I'd suddenly emerge, half-panicked, feeling an irrepressible need to move, to get out of the house, as though maybe by moving I could outpace this *thing* that had staked its claim.

And my mother would walk with me, and walk some more, holding my arm, saying little but accompanying me on my miserable marathon. I would talk and weep, and she would be there, just listening, trying to keep up with my race against losing myself altogether.

My parents lived on the ocean in an old shingled house that was and is a magical spot—eternally shimmering and summer-gold in my imaginings. My husband and I were married there; we'd spent Thanksgivings and Christmases and epic family gatherings of all kinds there. We would take our young kids on summer weekends to get out of the city.

But that particular August, it was cold and harsh, and my mom and I walked miles and miles of dreary coastline. I remember little but the urgency and the grayness, the cold mist on my face, and the simple fact of my mother beside me. I would come back exhausted, if not restored, and I'd retreat once again into my bed, curling myself tight with the blanket over my head.

What I didn't know then was that I'd only just begun my longest walk, the one that didn't stop when I returned to the house and dove under the covers. It was a journey I'd wake up to for days and months and years, and where it would land me I had no idea. My mantra was *I want my old life back,* but that was neither possible nor—as I'd only later appreciate—desirable.

~~~

The morning hours were always the hardest, the time when the terror made it difficult to breathe or move or even open my eyes. I remember waking in a fetal crouch, eyes clenched, both hands clawed tightly around my crotch, trying to displace as little air as I knew how. I downed the medication as soon as I got out of bed, but because it took hours to build up in my bloodstream, its levels were highest in the evening and lowest in the mornings—and my anxiety levels reflected those variations.

I was lucky in one important way: I never felt suicidal. But the places I traversed during that time were emotional hinterlands—at turns exotic and bleak and subterranean—places I'd never been and from which I wasn't sure I could find my way back. I felt trapped in an emotional labyrinth, so large and dark and byzantine it seemed to offer no way out.

But then, slowly, a month or so after beginning antidepressants, I started noticing I felt just the tiniest bit better come evening. A little less sleepy or wired, a little less out of control. As the weeks went by, this grace period started earlier in the day. As the levels of Prozac increased in my system, greater stretches of the day began to brighten.

I did still wake up in a panic most days. But I also remember—very clearly—the day when my mother asked if I'd like her to fix me a tuna sandwich for lunch. And I said yes.

Here's something else no one tells you: Recovery comes in hiccups.

Around the six-week mark, I left my parents' house and moved back home to Boston, a transition nearly as frightening as the early days after the breakdown. Fall was in the air. It was nearly time for the girls to go back to school. I was eating and mostly sleeping through the night. By then, my parents were emotionally exhausted. They'd never confronted acute depression before, and I knew that bearing witness to my suffering had been an ordeal for them. My husband arranged to keep travel to a minimum.

When I arrived home, everything was as it had been. The stoop was still there, the cats, the laundry, the kids still played and fought and needed feeding—and they were needier than ever. I was still scared enough to feel enervated, to need more sleep than I had ever needed in my life. Nearly every day for months and months, I found myself waiting for the bottom to fall out all over again, checking for that shadow just behind my right shoulder. At times I thought that I glimpsed it, obliquely, just biding its time—that I'd never feel safe again.

But, in fact, I did start feeling safer. The medication worked beautifully for me, and I found a great therapist whom I still see occasionally. I've never been able to come off the Prozac, and as much as I still hate to admit it, I'm probably a lifer. It may not be the recovery story some people want to hear, but for me, it's been one of the greatest successes of my life.

Because ultimately depression led me to writing—something I began to do at my mother's suggestion. Before my depression, I'd never written a creative word or really indulged in any artistic endeavor. It had always felt like too much of a personal risk. But having suffered such a profound loss of control, I found I couldn't go back to my old life.

Writing gives voice to the chaos and the beauty and the passion and the grief. It helps me to experience the world more deeply and to process what the universe chooses to throw in my direction. It's a joy so pure that when I'm unable to do it, I feel as if one of my hands has been lopped off, an eye plucked out.

When the writing isn't happening, I turn to visual art, another gift from my mother. These days, I spend long hours in my studio, fashioning art out of bits of paper and life's other detritus, making something out of nothing.

We're given only so many chances to feel and live at that volume. Despite the toll depression has taken—both on myself and the people I love most—it's allowed me to change the way I see the world and who I am in it. When I look to the future now, it's not a straight and predictable line. It's not a teary walk down a dreary coastline. These days, I rarely know what's coming next, and I can extrapolate myself in a thousand different directions that all make some kind of sense.

WITNESS

We haven't taken my eldest daughter to visit my brother in prison. We want her to remember him as Uncle Steve, not as Inmate 21368 at the county jail.

—Rebecca Schumejda

CONFINED TO QUARTERS

MARIANNE GOLDSMITH

First light, dim light, cold. Warming Jerry's right hand in my left, his rough, calloused fingers laced between mine. Moving in closer, we line up on the long, broad walkway, bordered on both sides by curved railings and blue garbage cans.

> *[1] Santa Rita Jail, aka the Greystone Hotel, is "considered a 'mega-jail' and ranks as the third largest facility in California." It is further distinguished as the first jail in the country to build its own smart grid. Visiting hours on Saturday for units 1–4: 8 to 11 a.m.*

We woke in the dark. Hot coffee, cold bread, sour breath.

> *[2] Visitors: Be there early or miss the first cutoff.*

I know women who spent time here years ago, political activists, arrested for protesting the Vietnam War. Some served time on weekends so they could hold on to their day jobs.

Not so for Daniel, son of Jerry (both pseudonyms), in November 2007. Off his meds, Daniel went to a bar, got spooked, and lost his temper. The man he injured has since recovered. Judge offered time in a group home, but Daniel said no. He's in jail for three months. Won't take his meds. He asked to see me.

This place looks like a suburban cinema multiplex, surrounded by walls of salmon pink and neat, tiered lawns of emerald green. Stadium lights on thin poles have been planted amid clusters of dark-red plum trees. Our ramp cuts through the middle, leading up to the entrance: an arched, white portico flanked by uniformed guards.

Jerry drops my hand, pats his jacket pocket, pulls out the sports page he grabbed just before we left. He grins, pointing to the cover shot, a quarterback caught in mid-air chase. He licks his lower lip, frowning, pulls out his handkerchief, blotting a crusty cold sore. He breaks out every time there's trouble with Daniel. When we married, my friends brought a housewarming gift and asked me what it's like to be a stepmother. "Look up," I said, pointing to fingerprints streaked across the ceiling. That was tall, long-legged Daniel, watching a ball game with Jerry, leaping, whooping to high-five the ceiling when his team scored. That was Daniel, before his break. Before college, too many drugs.

Last week, Jerry drove to Santa Rita, waited his turn, got all the way to the Mental Health unit, but Daniel wouldn't see him. Could happen again. Only now, we know better. Instead of instant panic over unanswered emails and phone calls, we can wait. If no one in the family, including his mother and brother, hears anything for 24 hours, we check his place. Longer than 48 hours, we decide whether to call the cops and file a Missing Persons report.

Our best teachers are the families in our support group. During the first year of Daniel's break, in the late 1990s, we faithfully sat in Thursday evening sessions, telling our stories, listening to theirs. Unless you were a "consumer" (patient), you could not give advice. We talked about schizophrenia, mood-disorder meds, side effects. We traded books and articles about mental illness. Yes, I got smarter. But I was still frustrated, furious with Daniel, watching as the disease bounced him around, in and out of paranoia, jabbering monologues, falling into sorry depression. I was frightened by how helpless and exhausted we were, caught up in this undertow.

Now, I watch Jerry move in and out of his own fog. He isn't ready to change his storyline for the child he nurtured with his ex, to let go of the bright wide-open world they wanted for him.

"Hey you," I nudge. "Apple?" I drop a slice of fruit from my bag into his palm. He kisses my hand, eats the apple, and goes back to the sports page.

About my dilemma, it's been long and messy, many fifty-minute hours sitting with my therapist, patiently pulling apart and putting back together what I can and can't do. What is out of my hands, irrevocable. I set up a separation, a kind of hyphenated space, between my life and Daniel's. From that place, I can see him.

Jerry says the deputies let in one hundred people at a time. From here to the entrance, I'd say we're about eightieth in line. I'm looking around at all the women here. Clearly, we outnumber the men. The younger ones look under or barely over twenty, Hispanic or African American. I watch them pacing back and forth, a bit wobbly, balancing on their toes in their high-heeled boots as they hover over cell phones. They wear butt-cheek-hugging jeans and short jackets with fur-trimmed hoods. Some mothers have brought their children, who tag after them, zigzagging, bopping around, staring at strangers, like me. Babies are bundled up in strollers or held over the shoulder, small sleepy faces yawning, peering out of bubble-gum pink or lime-green blankets.

> [3] "No food or drink is permitted in the visiting
> areas. Visitors will be allowed to bring one(1) dia-
> per and one baby bottle(1) into the visiting area."

I'm chewing on my sweet apple, surveying the crowd on the opposite side of the ramp. A set of regulars are camped out there, many settled in portable chairs, wrapped in fleece blankets, wearing thick socks and running shoes. Directly across from us, a woman sits wrapped up in red fleece with a textbook on her lap, highlighting text with a yellow marker.

A few yards ahead, two African American men in watch caps stand around holding coffee cups, shrouded in black-and-white

Oakland Raiders blankets stamped with the face of the team pirate, a player wearing an eye patch. One tall guy—he's got to be over six feet—strolls around covered in a pink Pooh bear throw.

"Why can't she give us something we need?" the woman in front of me, a middle-aged blonde, complains to her friend, an African American woman around the same age. "I put all that stuff from my mother in the closet. I swear, it's all brand new, still in the box. Waffle iron, blender, toaster oven."

I shoot a sideways look at Jerry, but he's still reading.

The woman is outfitted in snow-white running shoes and a turquoise velveteen jogging suit, arms folded across her chest, hands under armpits. "I keep telling her, 'Stop bringing us this shit.'"

"I hear you." Her friend nods and zips up her blue parka, shoving her hands in the pockets.

The woman carefully lifts the soft hood of her jacket up over the lacquered curls. Her cheeks are smoothed in rosy makeup, lips glossy pale pink, eyebrows surgically penciled in dark-brown strokes, eyelids shadowed, lashes stiff with black mascara. "I mean, who needs more than one toaster oven? I'm running out of room."

She kneels down to retie the laces on her shoe. As she straightens, she looks me over, my lumpy profile, black quilted jacket, floppy pants, flat walking shoes. We nod, trade smiles as if we were old friends. We know who we are, the women who show up. Whatever, whenever.

From my mother, I learned how to show up, the practice of *bikur cholim* (visiting the sick). In Jewish tradition, it is said, the visit removes a small piece of the illness from the afflicted. Would that it were so.

A trio of small birds hops lightly along the pavement. Seconds later, they're off, chased by wiggly kids pursued by mothers, mincing after them in their spindly shoes, weaving through the crowd.

Sky brightens. Doors open. Our line moves forward. A steady, rumbling noise comes from one of the camp chairs. Can't tell who is buried inside the dark hooded parka and blanket, snoring peacefully.

A deputy appears, making his way through the line, handing out forms. Jerry takes one, fills in the blanks with Daniel's name, his PFN—Personal File Number.

The huge lobby has high industrial ceilings, black-and-gray walls, and a gleaming white floor reeking of piney cleanser. Before I store my bag in a locker, I grab a smudged pocket mirror, pick at shreds of leftover apple between my teeth. I'm not surprised by my washed-out, freckled face, puffy eyes, but I pull out a tube of lipstick and dab a bit of coral over my mouth, grab my brush and run it through my hair.

After inspection, we pass through the metal detector and follow the crowd down a long beige corridor, under cold fluorescent light, until we reach the Mental Health pod. At the glassed-in booth, the guard takes our paperwork.

We're back to waiting with the others. I reach for Jerry's hand, and we slump against the wall. I notice a little round camera nestled above the guard station. Should I wave?

Jerry wants a good visit, a peaceful visit. He broods and grows snappy whenever Daniel lands in the hospital or goes missing. One night, I woke when I heard Jerry weeping, switched on the light. I rubbed his back slowly. He turned and looked at me. "I love my son," he said. "I don't know how to help him." Without his glasses, his blue eyes seemed so much smaller; he looked so defeated.

We miss the Daniel we knew, the sweet, depth-charging, wide-angle, whimsical explorer. What holds him unseen from us, in shadow?

On Saturdays, I go to the synagogue. During the Torah service, I stand when the rabbi asks for names of those who need healing:

> [4] *Prayer: May the Holy One overflow with com-*
> *passion upon him, to restore him, to heal him, to*
> *strengthen him. . . .*

After half an hour, the guards tell us they are notifying inmates of their visitors. I can't stand around any longer. I wander up and down the long bright corridor. Last time I saw Daniel, he was in court for his arraignment.

We take turns sending short letters and notes. Mine are basically weather reports, film or book reviews. Once in a while, Daniel will send a letter in penciled, jagged handwriting that makes sense up to a point, as if the writer had difficulty translating the news from too many voices talking at once.

On my second round of up-down pacing, I discover an interior window with a view of the visiting room. The space is divided into an open area for visitors and a row of three glassed-in booths, each with an empty chair for the inmate and a telephone receiver. On the visitor's side, there's a chair, a waist-high ledge, and a corresponding receiver on each partition wall.

Round three. I can see Daniel through the window, sitting behind the glass in the far left booth. He looks up and sees me waving. He tilts his head, gives me a tight, pained smile. He looks calm, clean-shaven: a buzz-cut scalp, his round face pale, his broad shoulders slumped in a dark-green uniform. I motion to Jerry, and he comes to the window, waves stiffly at Daniel.

> *[5] Advice: "Remind yourself that your loved one has an illness, not a character flaw, and it is not anyone's fault."*

We hear our names called. We push through the heavy door.

Jerry stands against the back wall of the room. I am seated at the booth. I raise the telephone receiver, looking into Daniel's dark eyes. As soon as we begin to speak, it's clear between us. We almost manage to cut through the glass.

Postscript: Ten Years Later

Hope comes in small doses. Jerry and I are sending letters to Daniel, who is back in Santa Rita with a broken ankle and serious felony charges.

We will visit him soon.

Sources

Note [1]: Quote and paraphrased summary from "The New Santa Rita Jail" and "SRJ Visiting Schedule," Alameda County Sheriff's Office website.

Note [2]: Based on advice for visiting inmates from an online chat room.

Note [3]: Quote from "Visiting Rules and Regulations," Alameda County Sheriff's Office website.

Note [4]: English translation from Jewish prayer for healing, *R'fuah shlemah*; see "Jewish Prayer for the Sick: Mi Sheberakh" by Rabbi Simkha Y. Weintraub, *My Jewish Learning* website.

Note [5]: Quote from "A Family Guide to Psychiatric Hospitalization," Depression and Bipolar Support Alliance (DBSA) website.

CAMERA OBSCURA

~~~

REBECCA SCHUMEJDA

Every science experiment starts with a hypothesis. I've proposed dozens of explanations and conducted subsequent investigations since the tragedy occurred, and still the truth remains elusive.

Yes, my brother has been incarcerated for killing his fiancée, but I'm not thinking about that now. Right now, I'm concentrating on the pinhole camera I'm helping my eldest daughter make for her elementary-school science fair. The construction is simple: a light-proof container with light-sensitive photographic paper at one end and a pinhole at the other. The process could be likened to the way a schizophrenic's mind works. There's only darkness, then the outside world invades through a tiny hole, and the mind takes what is there and flips it upside down.

I get the concept, but I really don't.

My daughter wanted to use her science project from last year, a homemade lava lamp constructed from a two-liter soda bottle, vegetable oil, water, food coloring, and Alka-Seltzer. *Come on,*

Mom, no one will ever know, she argued. *But we will, and why bother if you're not going to learn something new?* It's the fall of 2015, and we've just moved an hour north from an upstate city in New York with a population of 23,731 to this rural town of 1,469. She's adjusting. The bugs, the mice, the woods, the quiet nights creep her out. She constantly reminds us she hates living here.

His sons, my nephews, were asleep in the house when my brother Steve stabbed their mother to death a year ago on Labor Day weekend, but I can't concentrate on that. I've thought about that for hours, days, weeks, months; now, I'm focusing on what I need to set up a makeshift darkroom in our upstairs bathroom: dark curtains or maybe just black plastic garbage bags, a red light, and developing solution.

This project is becoming more complex than initially planned. There are so many steps. It's like trying to understand how someone you thought you knew could commit such a violent act. I went to seven different stores in search of black-and-white photo paper, and none of them carry it anymore. We finally sent away for the paper, which took more than a week and set us behind schedule. *Mom, if we lived in Kingston, we'd find the paper,* my daughter said.

Before the tragedy, if someone told me this could happen in our family, I would have thought they were insane. For a long time, my husband and I were convinced that someone else had done this and framed my brother.

On the side of my refrigerator is a photo of Steve and me from 2010. His arm is wrapped around my neck, his wrist rests on my shoulder, and his hand cascades over my heart. The picture was taken on Halloween in the kitchen of my old house, the house my daughter wants to move back into. She was dressed as a ladybug; she'd just turned two. She wore a pair of red rain boots, too big for her, so that when she walked, her foot slipped out and into a mud puddle. She would've finished her rounds with a soggy sock sloshing around in her boot if Uncle Steve hadn't taken off his sock and given it to her; it was ten sizes too big, but her boot didn't slide off again.

In the picture, we're smiling, my little brother and I; my head leans against his, or you could say his head leans against mine. Amy was there, too, the woman he says he still loves, the woman he killed four years later, even though she isn't visible. She was the one who told us to smile; she's the one who captured that moment.

I help my daughter, who's now eight, cover the inside of the box with black duct tape. She's singing a song about togetherness she says her class will sing during the morning assembly on Thursday.

I smile, because this is precisely why we moved here to this small town. My husband and I were exhausted by the negativity that permeated Kingston. A normal conversation at the bus stop between parents with young children in tow went something like this: *Yeah, he's with that ho, I'm gonna fuck that bitch up, show her what's up.* We thought we only had to protect our daughters from the outside world.

My childhood in the late 1980s was privileged in that my dad advanced himself from poverty to the middle class and took his family with him. He was a roofer in Long Island and embedded his work ethic in us. He never stopped, even after he was told by his cardiologist that he needed to slow down. There was a magic about him; he had this way of making people feel good about themselves, as if they could accomplish anything. He was my biggest supporter when I began writing.

In my seventh-grade English class, the teacher asked us to write a poem, but she thought my poem was too dark. She then summoned the principal, social worker, guidance counselor, and my parents to a meeting, where she expressed her deep concern for me. She actually didn't like me; I'd stood up to her several times in front of the whole class. She had a desk drawer full of Koosh balls—colorful balls made out of rubber strings that attached to a soft rubber core—and she'd toss them to students when she wanted them to answer a question. As I recall, she derived an unhealthy amount of pleasure from pelting daydreamers. Her cackle would permeate the room.

We all sat around the table. The teacher went on and on, the social worker chimed in, the principal advised my parents that the poem was a warning sign that shouldn't be ignored. My dad listened, and when his turn came, he asked to see what I'd written.

He reached out his calloused, tar-stained hand. The poem was passed to him, and the room went eerily silent while he read. My mom stared down at the table, as if she were the one on trial. I watched my dad's eyes move over my words for what seemed like forever. I remember thinking he'd taken time off from work just to read a poem.

After he was through, he tossed the paper down, put his gigantic hand on my shoulder, and said, *This is a really good poem, Rebecca, a really good poem.* For a minute, no one said anything, but then my dad looked directly at the teacher and said, *Don't ask students to write poetry if you don't want to hear their truths.*

A pinhole camera's shutter is composed of duct tape and aluminum foil; it opens and closes to expose the film. The shutter's purpose is to protect the film, just as a parent protects a child, as my parents protected us. But once the world comes spilling in, the parent doesn't have control over what happens to the child; outside forces come into play. With an old-fashioned photograph, there's the angle at which the camera is pointing, the intensity of the sunlight, the way the film is transported and handled, the chemicals used during the developing phase.

Although we were all thinking it after Amy's murder, one of my cousins was the first to say, *Thank God your father isn't alive. This would kill him.*

In the spring of 2015, the day I moved Steve's belongings out of his house pending a short sale, I came across some other faded family photos. I found these vestiges of my childhood a week after my mom was sitting in the kitchen of the parents of the woman my brother had killed, visiting with her grandsons. As she told me later, my mother was already feeling out of place when Amy's sister bluntly stated, *You know, he is going to spend a long time in prison.*

That's like saying, *You know, your sister is dead.*

There was no other reason for this statement but to inflict pain. For weeks, I was livid. Her statement was and is true. She had every right to be hurt, to be incensed; her sister had been murdered by my brother. I really liked Amy's sister before this happened. We weren't close, but I liked her. I don't dislike her now, but we are on opposite sides of a tragedy. If I were her, I would have said something even more incendiary to the mother of Amy's murderer. But now, all I want to do is ask her why no one wants to talk about mental illness.

My brother's body killed Amy, but his mind was not a willing accomplice that night. The evidence remains publicly undisclosed because he accepted a plea bargain, which spared him from a life sentence (instead he got 27 years in prison). So, the newspapers portrayed him as a monster who stabbed his fiancée to death, claiming the initial investigation showed there was a domestic dispute. But I've studied the evidence, and based on the limited explanations gleaned from police reports, forensics, and my brother's account, I've formulated my own hypotheses.

The day of the tragedy, Steve helped his soon-to-be brother-in-law work on his motorcycle, and then they decided to watch a football game at a bar. They drank at several bars until they were asked to leave one for being too loud. They headed outside, and then my brother bolted. Steve thought someone was chasing him. He said he'd been pursued by these people before and was terrified. He tried to get into a woman's car. He was screaming, *Help me, help me!* He staggered into the middle of the road and lay down. Another car almost hit him but swerved at the last second. Amy's brother and some other men pulled him to the side of the road, but Steve resisted; he thought they were going to kill him. He tensed up and tried to play dead.

My brother called a woman on the scene by his fiancée's name. He begged her, *Amy, take me home, I want to go home, I'm sorry.* When the police and Amy's brother came, the cops let him walk home with her brother; apparently, they believed the best remedy for too much alcohol was to sleep it off. According to the police reports, Amy's brother stayed for a while, waiting for his wife to pick him up, joking around with his sister for the last time.

No one knows the truth of what happened next but Steve. It seems likely, however, that not long after he was put to bed, he was spooked when Amy came into the room to join him. Later, he told a forensic psychologist that he was defending himself from demons—the demons none of us knew were haunting him. My brother chose to drink that night, even though he had experienced heightened delusions in the past while under the influence. He knew something was wrong but never asked for help.

I was two months pregnant with my second child when he killed Amy. My little brother got to hold my baby once, in the visiting room of the Madison County Jail a few weeks after she was born. He held her tightly against his orange jumpsuit, rested his nose on top of her head, and inhaled deeply until the guard stared at him. Then he handed her back, saying he remembered the first time he'd held his eldest son. We both teared up.

In 2015, after throwing out and giving away some of his belongings, my family carted the rest to the curb and put up a sign that read *FREE*; within a few hours, strangers had seized what was left. In one of the few photographs I kept, I was nine years old, and my brother was three; we sat sandwiched between my mother and father on an elephant's back. We were there at the same time in this picture; the circus of voices had not yet pitched a tent in his brain.

I often find myself taking the photo out of my wallet and turning it upside down, redistributing the weight, so that the elephant is crushing our family like mental illness has. I'm afraid of contributing to the stigma of violence and mental illness by telling this story—or that you'll think I'm trying to justify an inexcusable act.

In the county jail, my brother asked me to send him physics books, soft-covered because he couldn't receive hardcovers there. Before sentencing, he told me he looked forward to prison. Now that he was on antipsychotics, Steve said, he felt better than he'd ever felt before and that he would be okay, that we shouldn't worry. I was comforted by the thought of him working out equations for velocity, efficiency, and universal gravitation.

I'm afraid I'll never get the chance to hug him outside of a prison visiting area, while simultaneously terrified of the chance of hugging him on the outside.

But what I'm most petrified of is pretending this didn't happen.

After the photo paper arrives in the mail, my daughter and I go outside and set up the camera on a table behind the house. She hates facing the woods in our backyard because they frighten her. She pulls up the shutter and tapes it back. Then we go inside to eat grilled cheese sandwiches and chicken noodle soup, because the sun is shining but the temperature is below thirty degrees. We do this three times, exposing the film for different intervals—for thirty, ten, and five minutes.

Remember, I tell her. *If you expose the paper to light, the picture you took will disappear.*

When I was sixteen and Steve was eight, my mother swallowed a handful of pills. My father broke down their bedroom door and rushed her to the hospital, leaving us there. While I talked to my boyfriend on the telephone, my brother played with a toy fire truck, extending the ladder against the sofa, walking his fingers up the rungs to rescue the people trapped in a burning house. She was institutionalized for months, but we never talked about what happened.

In lieu of chemical developer, my daughter and I use a natural recipe we found on the Web composed of water, dried mint, baking soda, and Vitamin C tablets. Then we use water and lemon juice for the stopper solution. To explain alkaline and acid, we print out the pH scale and glue the pretty rainbow picture to her tri-fold display board.

In county jail, my brother was alllowed to have only four photos in his cell at once.

Sometimes at night, I sit on the staircase above the room my mom has stayed in since her son killed the mother of his children and listen to her cry. Every day, she asks, *How could this happen?*—the same way my daughter incessantly asks when we're moving back to our old house.

We can't go back, I tell them.

We try to help my mom. Last week, we urged her to connect with a therapist. She called Medicare and was told there was a one-year waiting list to see a psychiatrist. Nonchalantly, the woman on the phone told her that she could put her on the list if she wanted. *One year?* my mother asked again. *Well, yes,* the woman said, *at least one year.* My mother hung up.

When my daughter and I line up the three photos we took, from longest to shortest exposure, the images look like a row of waning metal bars.

After Steve had experienced several unusual incidents in college that we chalked up to binge drinking, my grandmother, my mother's mother, told me her husband had unexplainable episodes of depression and hopelessness throughout his life. My grandmother said he tried to kill himself a dozen times. Later, when I asked my mom about her father's episodes, she said she didn't remember.

The second set of pictures we took are close-ups of branches that appear to be knotted fingers trying to grip the empty sky.

I think of Amy, of the last day she spent with her sons, of the reverberation of her laughter. I imagine the terror of being ambushed by someone you trust in your own home.

We haven't taken my eldest daughter to visit my brother in prison. We want her to remember him as Uncle Steve, not as

Inmate 21368 at the county jail. We let her send him letters and pictures. He reciprocates with elaborate drawings and incoherent responses. He still sends letters and pictures to his sons, too, even though he knows I'm not allowed to pass them on to my nephews.

Until I could no longer close the lid, I stored them in a shoebox. Now, I place them in a plastic container. I wonder if there is enough space in my broken heart for twenty-something years of this.

I have a picture of Steve holding my daughter when she was a jaundiced baby. He's sitting in my grandmother's rocking chair, and she's resting on his chest. This had been taken only a few years after he left college. By the time my brother was eighteen, he'd been drinking heavily, but that didn't seem out of the ordinary for a college student. We'd had no idea he was actually throwing gasoline on a fire.

In the picture, my daughter's skin is the color of the jumpsuit he wears now. My brother looks down at her expressionlessly, as if he's cradling air. It makes me think of that poem I wrote, even though I can't recall what it was about. I remember how proud my dad was of my honesty.

The truth is, I don't care about the science fair. My hypotheses involve warning signs that could not have predicted what happened. I just want to prove to my daughter that if we're honest, we can, like light, travel through this tragedy as if it were a pinhole, free of distortion and manipulation—that we don't need to hide our thoughts in the dark chambers of our minds.

SACRED TOUCH

JULIE EVANS

I begin by massaging the tattoo on the top of his left forearm. I press my thumb on the upside-down *V* that precedes the number *72362*. Over the years, I've secretly jotted these numbers down a dozen times so they won't be forgotten. Through his stories, I see this man as the thin, pale fourteen-year-old Belgian boy he was the day he and his father were hauled away to Auschwitz. The story lives in his bones and his tissues. I read it with my touch every time I massage him.

It's 2016, more than twenty years since I met Jacob. In his late sixties then, he had suffered a stroke that impaired his right shoulder, memory, and balance. Now, he's close to ninety, a tiny man—4 feet, 9 inches tall—his feet so small (size 4) that his wife buys his shoes in the children's department. Still, he has the head of a grown man, a diplomat's face, mustached, bearded, and well lined.

His wife Hannah tells me she was born with "terrible bones," which according to Jacob, were made more crooked because nuns hid her from the Nazis in an unyielding wooden box. (I've changed both their names.) The first time I laid hands on her, she was 58 and had already had two knee replacements, two hip replacements, three cervical vertebrae fused, and an ankle fusion. She's bent and twisted, always in pain. I wish I could do what she asks: "Julie, just say *abracadabra* and make the pain go away." Abracadabra, my mantra now.

These days, Jacob and Hannah have me come once a week to massage them in their mountainside home just outside Woodstock, New York. She lives with scoliosis and osteoporosis and a husband with Alzheimer's. I have a new traveling table, heavier than the old one, so heavy I can hardly get it through my house, out the front porch, into the back of my truck, and into their house. It seems to weigh a million pounds. I'm sixty and sometimes think, "I'm too old for this." And then I remember what they've been through, and I lug my table up their cement steps, clutching the wrought-iron rail.

I've always begun by placing my hand over Jacob's tattoo as a silent prayer to honor what he's endured. Then I maneuver my fingers between his, willing the hard, stiff tendons to release so his hand will open all the way. Hannah begs me to get his fingers to straighten so he can once again do what he loves to do—tooling soft leather into high-priced handbags. I fight with his tiny feet to point and his toes to bend, so he'll have more agility to help keep his balance.

As my hands move through the massage, my soul moves through the story the body carries. I learn something new, and he can shuffle about a bit easier at least. He used to shower right after, but Hannah has him convinced it's best to leave on the oils and balms. For years, after the massage, the two of them, wrapped in their comfy robes, would putter around to make me an espresso, kissing each other like teenagers.

I've been massaging people since I was little, and now I've been a professional massage therapist for forty years. I grew up in Rochester, Minnesota, the home of the Mayo Clinic, where people from all over the world (and every relative I had, it seemed) would go for help. My parents were ill when I was a child—my mother an alcoholic, my father with severe emphysema—and being raised around pain and sickness taught me there's always something that can alleviate suffering. My dad used to say, "Leave a place better than you found it." I carry that notion with me everywhere. I take that thought with me when I visit the sick or care for the dying.

My parents died when I was seventeen, and they both died alone. I'm still sorry I wasn't there for them, but that sorrow became a calling two years later, when I got a job as a nursing assistant in a cancer hospital at the University of Minnesota. When people are sick, it's hard to think clearly and make good decisions. I learned by doing how to step in and get people the help or the love—or the touch—they need. I studied dying by taking care of dying people. I learned about death when I held the hand of so many as they took their final breath.

I'm a born-again Christian, a deacon in a vibrant country church, yet with Jacob, I don't know what to say to soften his resistance to hope. I have trouble finding words to encourage a man who watched as his father was executed. He can still describe seeing bodies stacked like firewood.

Once, when I asked Jacob if he prayed, he said, "To whom would I pray?"

I knew I was on thin ice. "How about God?"

"There is no God."

Those four words knocked the breath out of me—not because I'm so sure of what others should believe, but because without faith, I'm not sure how anyone survives.

⌒

The other day, Hannah waited for me in her blue chenille housecoat. She's so crippled now that she walks on the inside of her ankle bones. She's lost four inches from the scoliosis since I first met her. Her hair is white, and she's also lost too much weight.

"How has he been?" I hug her bony body into mine.

"Not good. It is never good. It breaks my heart to think of the man that he was." She has a thick Belgian accent.

"You're a good wife," I say, even though I sometimes have to scold her about yelling at her husband. She gets mad at him for not knowing to leave his walker in the doorway when he has to pee. She gets mad when he's confused and forgets what his sister's name is or where the kitchen is or how to drink a glass of water.

On my last visit, I noticed the bruises around her right wrist where she wears her Lifeline bracelet. "We fight," she said then. "He wants to get out of the house, and we fight."

Today, I massage her first, while Jacob lies on the couch near the fireplace, alternately watching us and dozing. When it comes to his turn, he's practically catatonic.

"He is gone," she says. "There is nothing we can do when he gets like this."

"I'll just massage him here."

I gather my creams and remedies, kneeling beside him. Hannah is right. He's gone. He doesn't respond in a way I can understand, but I hope that my touch will reach him. I start with the tattoo on his left arm and work my way from there. Alzheimer's may have taken his memory, but we can still connect in this way.

After years of touching the dying even when they can't hear or see me, I have to believe they still feel love through my hands. Touch transcends the other senses, especially when the dying have lost their mental moorings and themselves. For me, touch is sacred.

On my next visit, Hannah's arm is bruised and torn open. She says it's from her Lifeline bracelet digging into her during a fall, but I can see it's a bite mark. I put my hands on her shoulders and look her in the eyes. Her irises are a faded light blue; she looks so tired. She goes to check on Jacob, as I pull my massage table into the living room.

Hannah screams. "Come, Julie, he has fallen! I can't get him up."

It isn't a dramatic fall; he simply crumpled between an ottoman and a chair. But Jacob looks at me and says, "No!"

I'm struck stupid by this collapse. In hospitals and my private practice, I've seen many frightening things, and yet the image of this little man on the floor overwhelms me. Suddenly, I don't know how to be brave. Hannah has no balance or strength to help and just clucks like a nervous hen, staring at me, waiting, showing her complete faith in my choices. But for a moment, I don't have faith in me or in my ability to make a difference.

He weighs seventy pounds, the same weight Jacob said he was when he walked out of Auschwitz. His 87th birthday is just days away. I shimmy behind him, careful not to roll the leather ottoman into the huge TV. He's furious and clamps his armpits shut so I can't slide my hands under his arms. I'm stuck between a big leather chair and a fallen man with Alzheimer's. There is no give between his arms and the sides of his body, so I slide my hands under his diapered rump and heave him back onto the chair. He growls, "No!" again, trying to pinch me.

Good Lord, I realize. This is Hannah's *every* day.

Ten minutes later—though it felt like an eternity—Hannah unzips her thin housecoat and lets it fall to the floor, preparing for her massage. She grips my arm for balance. She stands crooked and naked in front of me, her body covered in bruises and scars. I unclasp the diamond-encrusted, heart-shaped necklace she wears. She releases the heavy watch from her narrow wrist and places it in a crystal ashtray on the end table.

She turns and looks me in the eye, shaking her head from side to side. "Oh, Julie. When I think of the man he was."

Her words move through me like heat. I don't say a word, but I do know the man that he was, as if it were coded in my hands.

For the hour I'm massaging Hannah, Jacob seems to be asleep in the big chair where I put him. Only once does he call out *Chou*, the nickname they have for each other. French for cabbage. He seems so alone, in a world neither of us can enter. Halfway through the massage, she confesses that Jacob bit her and she went stumbling into the kitchen counter. It's surprising she didn't break anything, but as I look into her tear-filled eyes, I see that something did break.

As Hannah rests, I go into the den to massage Jacob. I recount stories about his life that I've heard. I tell him how beautiful his home is and how well he takes care of his wife and son and two grandchildren. I brag about his huge success in the handbag industry. I laugh as I tell him how he and I both love to ride horses, but I never got to see him ride, that was before we met. His expression never changes.

But Jacob reaches out his hand to me. I take it. His eyes remain closed. He brings my hand to his lips and kisses it.

~

When I stop by to see Jacob a few days later, on a Sunday, he looks wonderful. The skin on his face is translucent; without his dentures, with his lips riding his gum line, he looks refreshed, as if he's facing something with new resolve.

Jacob is dying. It may be the only way relief can come. I've seen this look before in other patients, this temporary scrubbing away of misery. Sometimes, I'm the only one in the room holding some-body's hand when they exhale their last breath, but with Jacob, I probably won't be here. Just as I wasn't with my mom when she died of alcohol poisoning during our vacation in Greece, because the doctors had insisted I leave the room. Or when my dad died from pneumonia less than a year later, after battling lung cancer, because I'd left his side for a moment to use the restroom. Their sudden deaths—that permanent, gaping hole—nearly felled me as a teenager. Not being in the room when they died compelled me over the years to be there for anyone I could, although I've since realized I don't have to be the one physically sitting there. After decades, I've let myself off the hook.

The next morning, I can't get the image of Jacob out of my mind. I'm washing dishes, looking out my kitchen window at a deer standing in the lush field where my goats and little mountain pony used to romp and play. The doe stares at me the way she does every morning, after gobbling up all the bread I toss out for the birds.

I think of Jacob's cold, stiff feet. I uncovered them the day before, because that's what my preacher said he did for the dying. I've heard nurses on cancer wards say it, too. If you uncover the feet and crack open a window, the dying person's spirit can leave more easily.

On that last visit, when I tried to warm his feet, Hannah came into the bedroom with another visitor. There were already three other guests sitting in the living room, paying their final respects to the man who'd once been able to fix anything, ride a horse, wheel and deal, speak French—a man who loved oysters, martinis, the Mets, Belgian chocolate, fine wine. While I held his feet in my hands, Hannah and the woman approached his low bed.

They ignored me and murmured in French, clucking their tongues and shaking their heads. Jacob looked like a sculpture of himself, all bones and streamlined muscles. The skin on his face looked smooth, unwrinkled. He was curled on his side with full down pillows all about him. His hair had been freshly trimmed. I thought Jacob seemed like a young boy, maybe just before he was taken to Auschwitz, but Hannah said he looked awful.

The new visitor had big eyes and was about the same age as Hannah, maybe in her seventies, maybe more. She was obviously European, with well-coiffed hair and stylish clothes. She also seemed a little terrified. I suggested that we leave Jacob's feet uncovered, but Hannah insisted he was cold.

I wanted to find him a pair of warm socks, but instead I went into the kitchen. I busied myself slicing the thick chocolate torte I'd brought. I put out small dessert plates. Hannah came in and showed me where she kept the silver dessert forks. I fanned out five napkins beside the plates and put them in front of the other guests, who were now seated around the large dining-room table.

I was ready to leave, but the big-eyed woman reached for my hand.

"It's lovely that you could come," I told her. "It's a sacred time."

"No," she said in her French accent. "It is horrible. How could God let something like this happen to Jacob after all he has been through?"

"God didn't do this to Jacob." I tightened my grip on her hand. "Evil exists, but so does love, and love wins."

She didn't believe me, I could feel it through her fingers, but I didn't let go. I wanted to tell her that God is among us, working through us, that I feel goodness pour out of me when I lay my hands on people, and it doesn't come from me. Love is bigger than we know. It has to be bigger than Alzheimer's or the Holocaust. It has to.

I squeezed her hand a final time, said my goodbyes, and headed home.

⟜

This morning, as I stare at the deer, I call Hannah to see how Jacob is. I picture her picking up the phone in the bedroom, standing next to his bed.

"The same," she starts to say. Then she screams, "Oh, he is leaving now! Oh, Julie. He is going. Oh, Julie, my *chouki* is going."

And the phone clatters to the floor, and I hear her weep, and I weep with her. I feel the holiness of love creep into my bones. I hang up and watch the deer, who looks back at me one last time before leaping over the fence and disappearing into the woods.

LEGACY

And I think, who are these flower-worshipping, sauerkraut-eating people in my care? What can I do to keep them so strong, so resilient?

—Jamie Passaro

HOARD

APRIL NEWMAN

I never liked to let people know Eunice was my grandmother. She'd worn the same black curly wig since before I was born, and by the time I was twelve, it was mangy and patchy. Eunice's house in Dubuque—2792 University Avenue—was caving in, with its slumped shoulders, its red shutters like bloodshot eyes. It leaked and let in drafts and rats.

It seems like I'm exaggerating already, but I'm not. When I was eight, Dad and I used to take BB guns into her place and shoot them. Once, Dad shot a rat in the rabbit barn connected to her house. This was in the 1980s, when those *Ghostbusters* movies were popular. As a reward, Dad gave me a pin with a cartoon ghost that looked like the top of an ice cream cone. He proudly scribbled "Mousebusters" with a Sharpie over the side.

These days, I try to keep a safe distance from certain parts of my family history. I vacuum my floors. I reread Marie Kondo's *The Life-Changing Magic of Tidying Up,* watch TED talks on minimalism, and purge objects annually. I cannot explain exactly why this keeps me safe, but it does. When my scientist wife innocently brings home things she loves—baubles and beakers and test tubes to put on our shelves—or *another* kitchen gadget with the promise of more effectively juiced limes—I feel the walls caving in. I know how quickly an innocent Hello Kitty sticker collection can mutate into a full-blown hoard. When the garbage stinks of old sushi or expired milk, when there are piles of unopened junk mail on counters or clothes on the floor, I see all the things that aren't there, but are still.

⟶

Eunice collected and saved nearly every item acquired in her life, and entire rooms of her house were stacked full with boxes that held old clothes, china, faded flyers from my dad's bands from the 1970s (Trouble Bubble and The Hampton Road). She kept his cracked drumsticks, his childhood wrapped in plastic and fermenting.

By 1992, there was no running water or electricity in her house, which is why she lived in my dad's office next door and slept on a desk. And even there, she had no bathroom, so she peed in milk jugs. She wouldn't empty them out right away. She'd line them up underneath the window so the light coming in made it look like the jugs were full of apple juice. She smelled like piss and magazine perfume samples.

For much of the late nineties, Eunice could be spotted at a gas-station truck stop eating breakfast. She couldn't go to eat just any place; she'd been caught stealing food from buffets and stuffing cinnamon rolls and sausage links into her purse. She frequented the truck stop because they let her bring the dog. The dog was a collie, and as a puppy, he'd been a gift from my dad to me. But Eunice wanted him, so my dad took the dog back and gave him to her instead. I'd named the dog Charles after the Scott Baio character from *Charles in Charge*. Eunice renamed him Laddie.

There were other moments like these. Times when it felt like Eunice planted some hope inside me, then later took it back. Once, she brought me to a greyhound race, told me to pick the winner, and said if I was right, we'd split the money. After the dog won, I was thrilled and dreamed of what I might buy my mother, maybe a set of Eric Clapton tapes. But Eunice just kept it, saying *don't tell your parents*. For my twelfth birthday, she carefully wrapped a magazine insert for a year's subscription to *Spin* magazine. For months after, I walked to the mailbox, rain and snow. It was a year before my dad admitted she'd never even ordered it.

Dubuque was a small enough town for people to notice the stink of your unfortunate relatives. When calling friends in high school, I'd hear them bring up Eunice sightings as if she were a UFO. One of them wrote a punk rock song about her after I tried to describe that particular smell, titling it "Eau de Eunice." Before that, I hadn't realized my grandmother was something I should be ashamed about. After, I did my best to blend in, but by college, I moved away the first chance I got.

Eunice didn't seem so sick when I was a kid. I thought she knew rare secrets, like the fact that childhood was precious, which is why she had to save every artifact. Her house was rank even then, but to me, it seemed a marvel, a time warp. There was a secret apartment in the attic where her mother Augusta stayed until she died. Tiptoeing up the forbidden green stairs, I saw that the glasses were still dusty in Augusta's cupboard. An empty orange coffee mug sat next to the sink.

The adjacent room was filled with my dad's toys. There were painted cowboy figurines, a Western town set, and red plastic Indians. It was easy then, we had a shorthand—keeping these relics meant she loved being a mother the most. And as a child, that was so simple. The things she kept equated with how much she loved, and she loved larger than other people possibly could. I suspected I might, too. It felt so sacred that we had our own rituals. She'd heat one room with the fireplace and seal off the others with plastic; it was always cold. I could see my breath in the hall on the way to the bathroom. Everything was dark, painted blue, and I felt like a mermaid in some deep-sea cave on my way to Poseidon. She liked it when I told her so.

I could also follow her and hunt for objects or ride a scooter in the muddy backyard. She let me be my un-girlish self. In that hazy Iowa town, I got dirty looks for my sneakers. Or was told girls couldn't ride BMX bikes at the ramp. Sometimes I was mistaken for a boy. People were embarrassed for their error on closer inspection, but secretly I didn't care.

My dad became Eunice's favorite son after the youngest died in an accident. Mickey was his name, and he is forever eighteen years old in the pictures. From a clinical standpoint, it's easy to say the accident changed Eunice, earned her those addictions to Lithium and Salem 100's and objects, to so many *things*. That it was the stink of grief that clung to her clothes, but I can't know. To me, she was always the same mess of contradictions—a bottle of gin, a pack of cigarettes, a black wig.

She was candid about Mickey being her favorite. She wanted a girl to be her youngest, and Mickey let her dress him up in too-big heels and lipstick until he was in elementary school. She kept black-and-white photos of him in baby drag on the walls. On Christmases, her kitchen was too cluttered with junk for us to eat, and the living room had no free spots on the floral couches, so she put up the tree in her bedroom and insisted we open presents there. She'd point at Mickey on the wall, in his white dress, and remark, "Wasn't he a doll?" My father, mother, and sister crowded side by side, unblinking, but the way she spoke made it seem as if she'd opened her hands to only me—and there was a yellow canary inside.

I've heard this part of the story told and retold so many times by different people—whispered, the details mixing together like honey in hot tea—that it's become mine. Here it is now, mixed and contrived but the only truth I can imagine.

It's August 1, 1977, two hours after midnight, and my uncle Mickey is driving his Ford rough, knuckles pale on the rippled steering wheel. He has the eight-track jacked up with the Bee Gees to keep from sleeping. His chestnut hair is shoulder length, swooping up on the bottom like a woman's or maybe David Cassidy's. Mickey wears a thin gold chain around his neck and has no chest hair. The window is down, letting in the smell of lilies. He looks up in the rearview, sees the reflection of my parents' headlights behind. They're following in my dad's yellow Jaguar.

The roads are sloped like San Francisco's, and coming from the north toward home requires traveling up many hills. If it were brighter out, you'd see the white painted houses spaced very far apart and set back from the road; the patches of green lawns; the cars parked in driveways—the back of a Chevy Camaro or a Pontiac Trans Am. You'd hear my dad listening to Led Zeppelin—"Nobody's Fault but Mine"—as Mickey merges from Loras Avenue. He comes from University at the T-intersection with Westminster Presbyterian Church, which has a large limestone retaining wall facing the street and a white statue of Jesus above.

But Mickey doesn't notice this, because his chin is fading into his neck, and his brown eyes are glassy with drink. He doesn't bother to correct his arms, straightening the wheel after the right turn. He cruises into the lane of oncoming traffic across the yellow lines and stays the course. His eyes jar open only when the front tires mount the curb.

My parents see Mickey's red taillights bounce toward the telephone pole. And even though everything that happens next only takes about two seconds, time slows.

Mickey hits that telephone pole going fast, too fast. His head lolls to the side, over his shoulder and out the window before impact. He has all the time in the world to watch the windshield crack into slivers like an icy river. He sees it blow apart, the glass changing color from clear to tinted green and sparkling—an infinite number of pea-sized diamonds flying forward so slowly the stillness of night is reflected in each piece.

~

In my childhood, there was a way Eunice would gaze at his photos, then turn and talk to me—as if she were talking to him, as if something of Mickey had been born again in me. In her bedroom, I could dress up like a boy, putting on Superman shirts and capes. I could wear cowboy boots and vests and use my father's toy gun. I swelled with something like pride, which melted into shame as soon as I stepped off her front porch.

By the time I was in college, I stopped talking to Eunice. I discovered she'd put a number of cars in my name to avoid paying taxes. Her second husband got into an accident in one of them. (Not my biological grandfather, but the next guy, the one who was too tall and gray and looked like Lurch from *The Addams Family*.) She tried talking me into filing a false accident report to make an insurance claim. I refused. I wanted a regular life by then, one that conformed to the rules. A life with people. The cost of that was a life without her and, eventually, without my father.

When she died years later, in June 2008, my dad followed suit that fall. He was twice divorced by then, and just like Eunice, had started collecting cats. He'd even begun smoking. He and my sister were the only people to attend her funeral. After her death, he packed up a car and drove to Arizona, finally living out his cowboy figurine dream. He died in an emergency room with a cell phone that had no family telephone numbers stored in it, and he was buried in an unmarked grave.

With both of them gone, the City moved quick as a whip, seizing her property, plowing the house, dumping in backfill, and eventually extending the highway—rounding off the edges of her life and erasing the debris as a baker might with a layer of fondant. The neighbors were overjoyed. And with the tick of clocks and changes in seasons and technology running away with us all, the town forgot her.

But when I drive down that silky gray new highway, looking over the edge to the space that occupied so much of my childhood, I remember. The house with red shutters is now just an empty ravine, but it feels as powerful as an ancient leyline. We were hunters there, Mousebusters! I could be a boy or a girl under my red cape, and no one cared. There were pictures of me, next to pictures of Mickey. But there was always that smell, mold coupled with the sharpness of urine, and everyone ended up alone.

It's hard to breathe and drive now. It all comes as a wave. If I want to remember anything beautiful, I have to recall the ugliness, too. I do not get to pick and choose. My mind is too full, and I want to push this childhood away, which is easy because I'm stuffed with the detritus of my adult life. I need to call the handyman and fix the broken window, and there's mold in the bathtub near the grout, and the junk mail hasn't been shredded, and my skin feels like it itches—because of all the disorganized spice containers above the sink, the cups we don't use, the clothes that no longer fit.

And my heart starts to flap a little faster with these runaway thoughts, and I crack my neck and grind my teeth. The doctor says I should just run more, that if I did, I wouldn't need to take medication for anxiety. And it feels like weakness that I have to, but if running away worked, it would have worked by now. So, I make room for all of it inside. I look over the edge of the road and eat that space and swallow her house. I am like her and not her. Mickey is my spirit animal, the me-not-me who didn't live long enough to make a mess or clean it up, either. Eunice was outrageously cruel and incredibly kind, someone who loved too big but could not get beyond her own grief. And yet, she saw me as I wanted to be seen. It is, and I am, made of all these things.

NINE PHOTOGRAPHS

⟶

JOE VASTANO

It doesn't fall to the weak to invent myths.

When you have only shards of information about your origins, mythology works like mortar between the cracks to help assemble a mosaic that at least feels true. I invent myths about my mother Irene all the time—she took in stray animals, she ministered to the sick—but I'm careful not to assign attributes I don't actually see in her pictures.

Her sweet smile graces eight of the nine photographs my father gave to me as a child. She has light skin, a heart-shaped face, and big dark eyes. Her hair is also dark, relatively short and stylish—the way Jackie Kennedy wore hers. Her slight figure stands about 5'4", as compared with my father's height in the only photograph I have of them together. In it, they're dressed for a night on the town. My father smiles, his hand on the doorknob. My mother's head is listing a touch to her right, a dazed expression in her eyes and no smile.

In another photo, she sits on a couch with her hands laced together over her bare knees, revealing the delicate bone structure and sculpted arms she gave to me. She's one of the most hauntingly beautiful women I've ever seen, and I've known a few. She haunted my father until the day he died, in 1987, of heart attack number four.

But he was a ladies' man when they met in 1959, already married and divorced three times by the age of 32. Her eyes got to him, he said, the need for love and understanding he saw there. As he told it, their five-year romance demanded a lot of love and understanding—sometimes, heroic love and understanding—although no amount of either would have been enough to stop the tragedy that overtook the three of us.

He told me animals flocked to her.

One photo has her cheek to cheek with a lamb at a petting zoo, smiling like a child. Another depicts her hand-feeding a squirrel. I think my father took me to that same zoo when I was little so he could conjure Irene through me. He often said I was a carbon copy of her, which makes me want to remember how I moved before I had to cover it up with so many layers of tough.

I want the photographs to come alive so I can see us walking hand in hand to a school bus or her twirling me in the air or chasing me giggling around a yard. Sometimes, when I move my head a certain way or forget for a second how I need to look, I'll flash to one of those photographs and sense the very same movement from her.

Two of them contain evidence that I inherited her goofball gene. In one, she's stunningly dressed in a long, figure-fitting coat; a stylish hat; two strands of pearl necklace; black leather gloves and pumps. She poses like a model in front of a small pier in either Los Angeles or San Francisco, but undercuts her glamour with a smirk. My father wrote "Wow!" on the back.

The second is the only color picture, so faded with age it offers just a hint of hair color and skin tone. She stands on the shore of a Sierra Nevada mountain lake with her face toward the camera, dressed for cold weather in an elegant headscarf and coat. The hand nearest the viewer is in her coat pocket, while the other is spread wide over the lake. At first glance, she appears to be pointing to a family of ducks in the water, but she's actually showing off her pregnant belly—showing off *me*—her lips pursed in a smile that suggests she's about to stick out her tongue.

Maybe the reason there are so few photographs of her is that she ruined most of them by making funny faces. Like I do.

~

Whenever she was about to leave my father, she must have gotten a sign it was time to go, just as I did when I started disappearing from the lives of friends and family in my early twenties. I could always sense deep depression coming, like autumn's first chill at the end of summer. Like her, I always resurfaced, but only after I'd swung back to mania and could be the life of everyone's party again. In the meantime, I lived among strangers on the road, doing some form of outdoor itinerant labor and crashing on more floors and couches than I can count. Twice, I ended up in mental hospitals, just as she did.

Maybe we both felt invisible from the beginning, required to be happy little charmers no matter how sad or alone we felt.

From what I've been able to piece together, it seems clear Irene grew up in a family that routinely withdrew love for the slightest infractions. I imagine her escaping from that childhood, alone and acting out scenarios of being world-famous.

But more than anything, she wanted to be a mother.

My father claimed I was conceived because they felt their love was too big to keep to themselves. They both wanted me so desperately, he said, that my mother checked herself into a place he referred to as a "mental care facility" in order to get the psychological support she needed to carry me to term. He insisted that she could come and go as she pleased, and that they spent weekends together in the mountains during those months, staring into a campfire and dreaming of my arrival.

According to Mary, my foster mother, I was born a healthy baby, with sky-blue eyes she said entranced Irene. I like to imagine that everything about me entranced Irene, but she didn't get to be my mother for long. At the age of 26, she died a little over nine months later on December 22, 1964, from what Mary called "a brain tumor the size of a baseball."

The size of a baseball.

A baseball-sized tumor is big enough to eat half a brain, which makes me wonder where it started to grow. Did it suddenly short out the reasoning left hemisphere and throw her into the chaotic world of the right? That would indicate hallucinations to go along with her headaches. My father did eventually learn that she'd admitted herself to psychiatric wards when she disappeared. That sounds like hallucinations.

Two weeks after my birth, she deserted him for the last time. He found out later that she'd brought me to her mother's house in Los Angeles. My father figured she went back to try to heal the rift with her family; years before, she'd left her husband for him. I believe she was also thinking of a contingency plan—by then, she must have known she was doomed. But it turned out they wanted nothing to do with me, probably because I was *his* kid.

Their hatred of my father was so caustic they didn't allow him to attend Irene's funeral in south Los Angeles, which I assume was on Christmas Eve or Christmas Day. After they left, he told me he stood alone at her grave, holding an envelope on which he'd written "A Prayer for Irene, with all my Love." Inside was a letter he said he couldn't bring himself to read aloud:

> *My Lord, I wish to say something profound but I lack the education of words. I will simply say, take this loving heart to thy bosom and give her peace. This victim of circumstances who was torn between so many things. I know she tried desperately to find Thee. She had so much love in her heart that she didn't know where it belonged. She was a casualty of human suffering and her sensitive nature rebelled against the atrocities of life. I tried so hard to help but her affliction was beyond human endeavor.*
>
> *So I say to Thee, my Lord, take her and give her the love and understanding she so badly needed*

here on earth. I loved her so much, my dearest God,
and I will grieve for her all the days of my life.

    If Thou wilt do me the honor, tell her I will do
everything in my power to give her son all the love
and understanding that I know she would have given
him. I beg Thee to let us all meet sometime again.

                             —Joe

He'd intended to leave it on her grave, but he put the unopened envelope in his pocket instead, saving it for me.

I don't have a myth for why my mother placed me in a foster home before she died rather than with my father. The truth is, he drank and gambled and had already turned his back on four other children.

⟶

One member of Irene's family did acknowledge me.

Her sister Marie sent annual birthday and Christmas cards to my foster home in east LA, always with a five-dollar bill enclosed. No words, except for her name at the bottom and "love" written in front of it. I didn't even know who she was until I was nine or ten, assuming she was just another Okie relation of Mary's who figured I could use five dollars twice a year. Five dollars bought a lot back then: fifty candy bars or twenty comic books.

Marie called me for the first time when I was thirteen, not long after I'd been placed in McKinley Home for Boys in San Dimas, California. After some initial awkwardness, she started in on how beautiful, kind, and generous my mother was. I kept quiet, absorbing as much of Irene as I could, but Marie didn't get a minute into her tribute before she launched into a tirade about how evil my father was.

Blood is blood. I defended my dad, even though I didn't like him much at the time. Marie hung up and never called again. The cards stopped, too.

I wonder if my mother took Marie aside during her final months, begging her to give me the love she wouldn't be able to. The semi-annual cards were apparently the best Marie could manage. At times, I still wish I could have weathered her attacks on my father just to coax out a few more stories about Irene. Instead, I instinctively recognized another poisonous adult, and I've always been better off for that. My father may have visited me only a few times a year, but at least he claimed me.

As part of the GED exam I took at McKinley in the early 1980s, I was asked to answer this essay question: *Who would you most like to meet and why?* To my surprise, I wrote about Irene rather than John Lennon or Jim Morrison, two figures who were infinitely more real to me than she was then. I even joked about it afterward, telling people I'd passed the test because I made the grader feel sorry for me.

And yet, just a little more than a year later, I attempted suicide after I'd spent hours staring at those nine photographs, unable to conjure the slightest feeling for her. That led to my first 72-hour hold at a psych ward and the diagnosis of Bipolar 1, a biological gift from my father.

I spent the next two decades looking for her in the arms of almost every woman who offered love and understanding. In my late thirties, I started singing and playing Lead Belly's version of "Good Night, Irene" to the montage of photographs in my head. It seemed to narrow the oceanic distance between us to a river's wide spot. I could just make her out on the other side, smiling as she does in the pictures.

I got lucky and inherited her smile.

It's much more than a facial expression or a matter of identical bone structure. My mother's smile conveys the ability to seek and hold onto the sweet things in life between episodes of horrific mental instability. It's the single most important trait I got from her, and I hope she had no inkling I'd need to call on it so much. I hope she saw only how solid Mary was, how dedicated she was to her "brood," how crazy she was about babies. I hope she sensed none of Mary's joylessness and had no notion I'd be shattered by the loss of this mother, too. I like to think Mary reassured Irene as much as anyone could have during the last months of her life. Mary was good like that.

Perfer et obdura; dolor hic tibi proderit olim, a phrase from Ovid's "Elegy XI" in *Amores*, translates as "Be patient and tough; someday this pain will be useful to you." That works a lot better for me than the clichés people toss around about everything happening for a reason. When we grieve, we're not pining for the past so much as mourning the lost potential of a stolen future. I can't help feeling profoundly cheated that I didn't get a lifetime of sweet, tender, mysterious, classy, goofball Irene.

I wonder if everyone who's lost a mother at an early age thinks of her as a guardian angel. I know it was Irene who told my father to keep the letter he'd brought to her grave so I could have it someday. Years later, Irene whispered in my ear to stop drinking whenever I was in a black depression so that I didn't drink my heart blacker. I know she paced beside me, up and down the bleak hallways of mental hospitals, yelling loud enough to be heard through the Haldol so I could find a way out of there before it was too late.

NOT WHISTLING DIXIE

$\sim$

MAUREEN SULLIVAN

On the January afternoon of my fifteenth birthday, I came home from school to find that my mother had set the dining-room table with her rose-pattern silver flatware, gold-rimmed china punchbowl, and its matching cups, all arranged on a white linen tablecloth—a Dixie display of silver and status. It was 1978, when a peanut farmer was president, and I thumped up the steps two at a time to look for Mom. Our house in Dallastown, Pennsylvania, was empty-silent. The buzzing behind my eyes was not. I knew before I opened the bedroom door.

She'd left for Georgia while I was in school. She didn't leave a note, then or ever. She just left.

Dad didn't cancel my party. He put on his brave face while thirty kids spilled 7 Up and maraschino cherry juice out of the awkward china cups. I put on my normal face and smiled like I knew what normal was.

"Mary Ann had to go south to take care of her sick mother." That's what Dad said to the parents as they showed up at our door. Maybe we should have told them the truth, but we could barely tell it to ourselves. After that, the word *south* spit off my tongue and sounded vulgar and profane. Yet during our Savannah visits, the hushpuppies, fried shrimp, and sweet tea slid effortlessly down my throat.

When I discovered the unused Jean Naté bottles under her bathroom sink, I might have thought in a wishful instant that her leaving was retribution for the present I'd given her every birthday, Christmas, and Mother's Day. I'll never know what story my mother told herself when she pointed the Buick south and left on my birthday, but I know the story I told myself, and it was a doozy. It's taken me a lifetime and part of my daughter's lifetime to un-tell it.

⟜

My first parent-teacher conference fell just after the start of the twenty-first century, when we lived in the Pacific Northwest in a town called Battleground, named for a battle that was never fought. Miss Katherine beamed. She told me that in ten years of teaching preschool, she had never encountered a child as bright as my daughter. Olivia, she said, understood concepts a lot of seventh-graders struggle with.

I'm certain my face contorted into a near replica of Munch's *The Scream*.

What mother doesn't want to hear that her child is exceptional? Every mother except me. I was swamped by the thing I'd tried to ignore most of my adult life: the Southern crazies—the kinfolk on my mother's side—and the fact that their DNA could be loitering in my three-year-old daughter.

I thought of my toothless, jobless, bipolar, schizophrenic Uncle Billy, who—according to family lore—had an IQ of 210. *Higher than Ein-damn-stein* was how Aunt Margie put it. Billy lived with my grandmother in Savannah until she died. Then he moved to and got thrown out of and back into public housing until Y2K came and went without a catastrophe (unlike Billy).

And there was my brilliant bipolar mother who, after she'd divorced my father and stopped drinking again, moved into my grandmother's converted garage until she got married to her high school boyfriend. He hadn't been drunk in twenty years, but in less than one year with my mother, he was drunk again.

Miss Katherine's confusion was palpable. I half-chuckled and told her, "Oh, it's just that every extremely intelligent person in my family has been an utter failure at life."

My forced smile must have contradicted the panic I felt pooling in the corner of my eyes. "I'm not that smart . . . not enough for her."

"Maureen." Miss Katherine looked across the miniature table, where we sat like giants. "She has you. You love her, you'll keep her grounded. It'll be okay."

She smiled matter-of-factly, as though she'd settled it, then showed me some of Olivia's drawings. I could only nod and was still nodding when the next mother walked into the room.

What I really wanted to know was if I could be a good mother to my daughter. I wasn't sure what a good mother looked like. I wasn't too sure, either, what constituted a good daughter.

A good daughter doesn't fall asleep hoping that in the morning she won't have to step over her mother's body at the bottom of the stairs or that her mother won't have driven into the center of their small Pennsylvania town wearing nothing but a sheer nightgown to demonstrate how much she hated the North, the cold, damn North.

A good mother doesn't get so tanked at her own party that she forgets that the only sober guest told her he caught her daughter in an upstairs closet with her friends, drunk for the first time at age ten.

A good daughter doesn't wake up with a bruise of her own handprint on the inside of her thigh, because even in sleep there is little relief, and fetal-curling is how you cope.

A good mother doesn't paint over every Christ image hanging in your Catholic home with Latex White while you're at high school. She doesn't put your second-grade silhouette over the newly whitewashed replica of Rubens's *Madonna and Child*. She's not splayed on the kitchen floor drunk, psychotic, and paint-splattered when you arrive home from swim practice ten minutes before your date—a cute Mennonite and captain of the wrestling team—is due to show up at your front door.

A good daughter doesn't learn to forgive all the wrong people for all the wrong reasons.

A good mother doesn't throw heavy ceramic lamps at your sleeping father's head and then tell you to go to hell with a vacant, defiant gleam in her eyes.

A good daughter doesn't ever tell.

〜

Not long before that parent-teacher conference, a pseudo-friend complained about her crazy Kentucky relatives shooting squirrels out of neighbors' trees from the back porch. I assumed the squirrel story was a warm-up for the *real* crazy and thought I'd found a kindred spirit. I confided that I had Southern relations with bona fide diagnoses and told her about Mom's most recent lark of walking down Victory Drive in Savannah wearing nothing but a paper-thin nightgown. (Note to self: Send Mom some *solid* cotton pajamas.) I explained that my uncle had done the very same "victory walk" butt-naked ten years prior. *Ha ha.* I waited for her to one-up me, but she just shifted her spine and stared at my reddening face. I knew then I could one-up Miss Kentucky all damn day.

"My momma's people *win* at crazy," I said in my best Southern drawl. "Victory is ours."

Turns out, there's more than one kind of crazy, and my kin's crazy is the kind that frightens people . . . away.

But most of the time, I refused to own my Dixie heritage, so I was shackled to it, forced to repeat the blunders of my Rebel relatives. Easy mistake—my father was born in Boston. I was born and raised a Yankee in a dot of a place only half an hour from Gettysburg and, damn it all anyhow, you can't get more Yankee than that. I. Am. Not. A. Southerner. No, ma'am, I'm not crazy, only related. I put my useless fingers in my ears and *la la la*, but I hear my aunt's voice inside my head, her deep drawl, over and over, "Reeni-bean, just because you wish things a certain way, it don't make them true."

I was still fighting when Olivia was born. I brawled against the divided and delusional battlefield of my mother's brain like my relatives who still dispute aspects of the Civil War. I thought I was better off without facts. I believed that the geography of my birthplace was all that mattered, was what made me a Northerner, was what made me sane. I know now that my Southern mother could have raised me on the North Pole among elves, and I would still be more Southern than a child raised in Savannah by Mrs. Claus. But when I became a mother, I still needed to believe that I could secede from my past. I had good reasons. We all do.

⟜

Bipolar disorder is a mean, lonely, lifelong disease. I don't care what the textbooks or websites declare. Nothing and no one, not one drug, not one person, could keep my mother suspended for long in a state of equilibrium. My father was loyal to the core, and I don't doubt she loved him, but once her mind slipped off balance, it turned him and anyone else trying to help her into an ogre. To suggest her lithium levels were off when she cleaned the baseboards with a toothbrush for the second time in a day was like offering the cowboy with the biggest buckle at a rodeo advice on riding bulls. Drugs only work if swallowed, and sometimes not even then.

The disease divided my mother from her right mind: the kind, fun-loving, and generous mind that allowed her children ice cream with gobs of Hershey syrup every night before bed, when her eyes radiated tangible joy in the black-and-white pictures of her hugging us. Her disease and our shame separated each one of us—my brother, my sister, me, our father—from her, from each other, and from any chance of having a community. No one brings chicken casserole by if you don't mention that your mother is in the hospital getting electroconvulsive therapy.

I learned early in life how to lie, mostly by deleting the truth, mostly the honest and best parts of myself. As a child of the North, raised by a Southern mother, spoon-fed lessons on etiquette and status, I learned how to live my lies with gumption. "I'm just fine" is what I'd tell anyone who asked, no matter how far from fine I stood or knelt or crawled.

Because my mother's depressions ended with her in the psych ward at York Hospital, feeling slightly sad terrified me in the same way feeling remotely Southern did. When the inevitable and many griefs of life arrived, my "normal" depressions (I took a quiz on *Psych Central*) lingered longer because I sought no refuge. When I thought about suicide for the first time last year—and then continued to do so two or three times a day for months—I told no one, not my therapist, not God, not my dogs, not even myself. For long stretches of my life, I pretended . . . until I couldn't.

⌒

At the end of Olivia's eleventh birthday, after the homemade banana cake was put away and the ice cream was back in the freezer, my daughter asked me what I did on *my* eleventh birthday. I sat on the edge of her bed and came up with nothing—no image or smell or remnant of a memory. When I told her I couldn't remember, it wasn't a lie; it was an involuntary deletion.

Eleven was a bad year. I returned home after my first week away at Camp Cann-Edi-On, a scant half-hour drive from home, during the summer before I entered sixth grade. Mom was slouched and sniffling in her harvest-gold La-Z-Boy. The woman who'd driven me home walked into the house behind me. Mom blamed her runny nose and bathrobe attire at two in the afternoon on a lousy summer cold.

The other mother didn't stay to chat like mothers normally do. Instead, she softly shut our front door as though trying not to wake a baby or a giant. Through the deep underwater quiet of the house, I moved toward my mother and handed her my card of a daisy made with construction paper and glue so thick it was still drying. In my mother's hand, the card looked wrong, the petals too crooked, the flower too small, and I wanted to snatch it back, to make it better, to make the card into what she needed. I wanted to tell her about archery, canoes, and the god-awful food, and how I missed her cooking, but I just stood next to her chair.

My mother gazed through me, as though some faded movie in a faraway land was playing beyond my skull. She spoke, but the flat tone of her words offered no comfort. Her eyes were gone. Their utter nothingness swallowed the air around me. There was only her. I disappeared like the smoke rising to the nicotine-stained ceiling above her gold chair. The only movement in the room was her ashes dropping and me falling into a void of perfectness and people-pleasing. *Please. Come back, Mom, please. I'll be good.*

I wasn't ready to lose Mom. I couldn't face the truth, so I didn't face anything. My momentary awareness ended the childhood but not the child. The forgotten days at home stretched to weeks, then to months after I returned from camp, and to this day they remain blank, soundless, gone. If those memories are with me now, they're scribbled in a secret kid-code I can no longer decipher.

Days before my eleventh birthday, my mother was diagnosed and got her second round of ECT. If I could shake my eleven-year-old self awake, I'd tell that child to believe what her mama always said about everything: This, too, shall pass. I'd tell her don't shut down and attempt to please a thankless, normal world. And treat your body like you believe it might live past age 25, because 55 is not feeling so good.

The day after Olivia asked me about my eleventh birthday, I called my older brother and sister and asked if they remembered how we functioned as a household each time Mom left us. Didn't Dad work long hours? They couldn't remember, either.

⟳

I'm not proud of the fact that I was peeved with my mother when she died thirteen years ago, but I don't berate myself over it anymore. I've forgiven her for her unintended transgressions and absences. She always came back, and that counts for something. It has to. On a daily basis, I forgive myself for being so unforgiving, which is so Southern-polite of me, like sending a thank-you card for a thank-you card.

After you? No, after you. After you, Mom, because on some birthdays, I still chase after you.

Three years ago, when my daughter turned fifteen, she had a small party with friends who, like her, are more self-aware and informed than I may ever be. Today, the kid is okay. Matter of fact, she *is* just fine. She knows most of the story of my past, her past—not all, but I'll tell her when she's ready. She is kind and, like her father, has a high aptitude for forgiveness. I'm lucky. We have moments—normal, I'm told—when in her adolescent eyes, I can't do or say or be anything worthwhile. Some days, a look is all it takes, and I descend into my eleven-year-old self. Then I fight my way out of that lost place, into my body, into my backbone, and I mother her.

Poor kid is stuck with me and all the mistakes I'll make, but leaving my life, my daughter, my chance to heal her past—*God willing and the creek don't rise*—won't ever be one of them.

DISPATCHES FROM THE LAND OF WELL

~~~

JAMIE PASSARO

My memories go like this. I'm sixteen and driving Mom two hundred miles to Seattle for a psychiatrist's appointment—me at the wheel, because she gets panic attacks driving faster than thirty miles an hour, which is all the speed she needs in our town. And then we're shopping and shopping and buying lattes and shopping some more, thrilled to have made it, to have navigated that big city with its scary hills, both of us working the stick shift and the emergency brake of whatever sports car Mom and Dad are driving then, me revving hard, peeling out, doing what I can to move forward and up and not roll back into someone's BMW. Both of us laughing. A little Cheetos dust caught in her lipstick at the corner of her mouth.

She's recently dyed her hair, which was the same mousy brown as my hair. It's platinum, and it makes her eyebrows look very dark. In Seattle, she buys me a black-and-cream wool coat and a matching hat, flowered silk pants, and a cashmere sweater with embroidered flowers, all of it impractical for a girl in high school in a town with the most rainfall of any place in the continental US.

I've said I remember the waiting room of her psychiatrist's office more vividly than any of the bedrooms of my childhood friends, and this is true, but what I remember most from those trips is the shopping. I'd get euphoric just walking into a mall with her—a mall being an exotic place, given that the nearest one to our town, Forks, is three hours away in Silverdale. It's thrilling to be with her when she's excited, to know we'll buy a new outfit that day with matching accessories.

I wonder if these were manic times or just plain happy times for her, for both of us. "Manic" wasn't a word I would have known then. I still don't know, looking back, what was *too* up, though down—*too* down—those times were unmistakable.

This goes for both of us.

Now, it's 2015. I'm a grown-up at forty, though I'm still vaguely bemused with myself when I go to a meeting or rent a car. Like recently, when I drove to the ninetieth reunion of my college newspaper at Pacific Lutheran University. Two-hundred-and-fifty miles north, and the freeway exits were familiar, Sleater-Kinney, Pacific Avenue—*Pac Ave*. I was trying to remember how I started, what it was like when I didn't think I could have her illness, when I was nineteen and ate Thai food for the first time and saw Jewel live.

My friend from the newspaper staff and I went out for dinner at an old favorite restaurant, ordered the same thing we'd always ordered, talked about our kids, our husbands, our work. Then we went to the reunion, where there was no one we knew except for our newspaper advisor, who looked exactly the same, who was supposed to be retired but kept advising our old newspaper, the *Mast* (now folded into the digital *Mast Media*). He continued to rage about the typo in the headline at the weekly huddle, kept on sending those poor kids to cover the Board of Regents meeting. He told me he was also teaching a class on global ethics. I tried to think of something to say about global ethics, but could not.

I might have been projecting, but I felt he was disappointed in me for not sticking it out in journalism. It reminded me of when I was news editor and took off for a few days to celebrate my twenty-first birthday with a boy whose accent I liked very much. "Where have you been?" my advisor had scolded me when I returned.

Where have you been?

It's a fantastic question to ask myself. I am newly better after a long, fragile crazy. How I know I am better is that if I hear a siren or a train whistle, I don't think it's connected to something I've said or done. That car alarm, for instance, has nothing to do with the fact that I've left the kids alone in the bath to check my email for the forty-seventh time today. I can go out to a restaurant and no longer think the people at the next table are sending me messages in their sentences about how vain and self-absorbed I am.

I wish I were joking or exaggerating. It was a long two years.

What is good: full nights of sleep, my daughters' laughter, making dinner with a dandelion tucked behind my ear, the college radio deejay who just the other day played a Mozart concerto followed by "Rock Me Amadeus" by Falco.

What is bad: lost time, lost friendships, the possibility that the paranoia will come back.

Coming out of it is like emerging from a bomb shelter where I've been waiting with dread for months and months. And then, whoa, it's bright out there! And there are people and emotions to reconnect with, foods to taste, books to read, music! There have been four times now, four episodes, as they say, and each time my reemergence is tentative and sweet. Each time, I come back a little more vulnerable.

The other day, during a walk between winter rainstorms, my daughters and their friend dropped to their knees in wet grass around a budding crocus and began to sing a song they'd learned from their Waldorf preschool: *Crocus, crocus, waking up, catch a sunbeam in your cup. . . .*

It was charming—one of those moments as a parent when you watch your children engaging in something that's their own culture, completely separate from what they know from you. Like when they agreed they both loved sauerkraut, and one of them said she'd made sauerkraut before. And even though I've never made sauerkraut, it's plausible that somewhere in her eight-and-a-half years she has. And I think, who are these flower-worshipping, sauerkraut-eating people in my care? What can I do to keep them so strong, so resilient?

Last winter, I helped write the obituary for my uncle, whose heart gave out. I've always said I'd love to be an obituary writer, but I didn't realize how hard it is. You take a life and boil it down into a few salient grafs. He was a computer programmer and a poet. He was great with kids, lousy with money. He stood at his wife's funeral and rocked gently while they piped in Cat Stevens's "Hard-Headed Woman." I don't think he ever got over losing his wife, Julie. He took good, fierce care of his son, my cousin, who has schizophrenia. He called me "Jamikers" for my whole life. I Googled his poems, and they're pretty good. I like the one where, house in foreclosure, he took off to Maui for the wedding of a distant friend, ended up teaching some of the other wedding guests to body surf, eating Thai brownies and drinking mimosas with them, remembering that "making new friends is one of the best things."

I always remember compliments. My uncle came up to me at my mother's memorial five years ago and said I'd "killed it" when I spoke. I had listed her favorite things, such as giving gifts and Nordstrom and high-thread-count sheets and Ellen DeGeneres and that moment when you sit down at the restaurant and they bring you the basket of bread.

How she could rip off the price tags from a new item of clothing so stealthily with one quick snap, they'd be in the garbage before you could open the drawer to get the scissors. That song she had as the ringtone on her phone, "Bad Day" by Daniel Powter. I talked about her acceptance of some of our differences, how she endured hundreds of vegetarian dinners and even ate Tofurky one awful Christmas, for Christ's sake. How she handed over a Chevron card for a cross-country trip I took when I was nineteen, even though it must have scared the shit out of her for me to be traveling that many miles alone. You can pretty much live on the food you buy at a Chevron gas station, especially when you love Diet Coke and soft serve and Red Vines, and she never did question how much I spent on "gas" that summer.

When I was eight, a Seattle TV crew came to interview us for a feature about Mom on a magazine-style show, when everyone thought she had miraculously recovered from her illness that never had one name, that had, at times, manifested in a mom who didn't want to get off the couch. She'd recently traveled from our home on the Olympic Peninsula of Washington to Boston for an experimental surgery in which a neurosurgeon used lasers to try to zap the depression from her brain. Some other doctors were critical of the surgery, calling it witchcraft, but for her, it was a success at first.

I don't know how much of that success was a placebo effect or how much was temporary relief from the otherwise unstoppable depression that gripped her brain, turning her from sunny to flat. I don't understand her illness now, and I for sure didn't understand it then. But at the time, at that moment, from the TV reporters' perspective, it was a story with a happy ending. I can picture the cameraman filming me swinging on my rusty, creaky swing set as the sun filtered through the tall Douglas firs in our backyard. A reporter asked me if there was anything I wanted to say about my mom. Even at that age, I felt pressure to say something interesting, but I blurted out the first thing that came to me, maybe the truest thing: *I want to say that I love her.* That's how they ended the segment, just my voice.

Mom and Dad didn't want me to appear on camera; I'm not sure why. Our town was so small and isolated, anyone who saw the segment would know the voice belonged to that well-dressed Anderson girl with the bowl cut and the buck teeth. *I want to say that I love her.*

We had wiener winks for dinner the other night. These are hot dogs with cheese broiled on bread and served with ketchup and relish. Only we use veggie dogs because we're vegetarian. Ga-Ga used to make these, I said to the girls. It's a reminder that I had a mom who died, and maybe it's also a story about how Mom didn't cook. Except that she did, every night for years and years, dinner with a side salad of iceberg lettuce, tomato wedges, and Thousand Island dressing.

If I had a sister, she would say to me, *Remember the lasagna, remember the meatloaf with the bacon on top?* And I would say, *Remember how she used to leave the spaghetti out on top of the stove overnight?* And the sister would say, *Remember how she used to make those bar cookies in a nine-by-twelve baking dish, and they would sit on the counter with a butter knife in them, and you could just walk by and cut yourself a rectangle anytime you wanted?*

And I would say, yes, she used to make the bar cookies when she felt like a sweet but didn't have time to spend on cookies. And maybe then we would remember the times she would make a small impromptu batch of cookie dough in a measuring cup, egg and all, and we would eat it with a fork.

I want to say this is how we remember. I wish I had a sibling to do this with, to help hold accountable my memories and sort out what was the illness and what was Mom's quirky personality. Mom's depression developed after I was born, and she was in and out of hospitals for years, so my parents didn't have other children.

I was always caught off guard by Mom's illness, by something that was such a fact of her life that we hardly ever talked about it. Now, that seems astonishing. And maybe not astonishing. If she hadn't been so adept at coping, maybe we would have talked about it more. Maybe we would have had a protocol or a system, but that's hard to imagine. In times of wellness, were we, her family, really going to come up with a contingency plan for if she thought the telephone wires had messages for her? What if she thought people were tiptoeing past the house at night? What if she wanted to launch a business selling soft biscotti to the masses, as she did in the last manic-y months of her life?

When you're well, it seems to me, in her life and in mine, what you think is, *that part of my life is over; I'm solidly living among the well.* You don't want to come up with a contingency plan, because you're sure there is no need.

When you're unwell, in her life and in mine, denial is a reflex. The alternative is a long set of appointments and the meds with the creepy side effects like drooling and shaking and eating M&Ms by the bucketful and maybe a trip to the psych ward and all the dealing and the help-talking and the facing up to not being okay.

I have been in the thicket, and I have been outside the thicket calling in, when it seemed that we, the people in Mom's life, were going to let her down either way, by overreacting or underreacting to an episode. Is that the way it was, or is that what I tell myself? Is that what people tell themselves about me?

I'm at a steady place now. Maybe that's tenuous, if you study the narrative. I can still conjure up what it was like. I watch a red car drive by my house or read something in a magazine and know that just a year ago, I would have thought the car was a sign or that the words in the magazine were speaking to me in some way. I shake my head hard to physically dislodge the thoughts. I wish I had better armor—like my dad, who, after a serious car accident, bought himself a Chevy Suburban. I think that's what we all do—protect ourselves in the best ways we can from what we know from our pasts.

What I know is that if Mom were here, she could meet my second daughter, who looks like her in some ways—same blue eyes, same big smile, same blonde hair. Which is funny, because Mom had dyed hers for years. Viv is ebullient, like Mom was when she was truly happy—baking with my first daughter, Olive, right before the start of the movie or when Dad came home from work or when she bought me a new sweater.

Viv, at five, asks about *my* day, just like Mom would. But Viv's laugh is something all her own. She throws her head back and busts up, staccato laughs on laughs, harder and longer and more joyfully than any of us. Mom would have loved to hear it.

EPILOGUE

*We all resist the notion that life is a series of scat-
tered moments. Light does occasionally dawn inside
our skulls, but then the darkness comes down again.*

—Martha Nichols

WHY GOING CRAZY
ISN'T JUST A GOOD STORY

MARTHA NICHOLS

I will always love good stories, the ones that take you on a rollercoaster journey of emotions, revealing recesses of the human heart. I'm a writer and a teacher of writing, and classic narrative structure is seared into my skull—to borrow an image from Mary Karr, creator of such literary rides as *The Liars' Club*, *Cherry*, and *Lit*.

When it comes to memoirs about mental illness and addiction, though, I've grown suspicious of "good stories" in recent years. Their controlled narrative arcs seem worlds apart from what I experienced when visiting my aging, bipolar mother in the midst of a mental breakdown.

Terrified, she would bombard me with stories of the most dramatic kind—raw, metaphorical, taboo-breaking—but they changed each time she told them. During a visit with her not long before she died, this thought came to me like a sudden punch: *Maybe nothing she's ever told me is true.*

As much as I've appreciated mental-illness-related memoirs by writers like Karr, William Styron, and Martha Manning—they've been touchstones during my own brushes with depression as well as my mother's episodes—there's something about the neatness of their structures that I don't trust.

I feel this way even about one of my past favorites: *The Eden Express*. Mark Vonnegut, son of the famous Kurt, wrote his first "memoir of insanity" almost four decades ago (it was originally published in 1975). While I still appreciate its many strengths, I no longer fully buy into it.

Fortunately, Vonnegut's 2010 sequel, *Just Like Someone Without Mental Illness Only More So*, continues his story past a traditional happy ending. When it was first released, *Publisher's Weekly* called the book a "slightly subversive memoir." I wouldn't say "slightly." One of the many pleasures of his wryly titled second memoir is that it exposes conventional recovery narratives—including Vonnegut's earlier one—for what they are: tales that have been massaged for dramatic impact.

I remember inhaling *The Eden Express* in the late 1970s, gripped by its powerful narrative: young Mark, trying hard to be a "good hippie," lighting out for British Columbia with college friends to live on a commune—and ending up hospitalized during the course of three psychotic breaks.

Psychosis doesn't lend itself to linear plotlines, but *The Eden Express* follows a familiar story arc. There's the lead-up to the crash, with poetic forebodings or just plain weird behavior. There's life on the ward, complete with comic fellow inmates, clueless psychiatrists

(Vonnegut describes "Dr. Dale" as having "the emotional depth of a slightly retarded potato"), and moments of connection with Somebody Who Understands ("Dr. McNice"). There's the slow recovery that makes the sufferer wistful but wiser.

Reading this story again more than thirty years later, I'm struck by the benighted attitudes toward mental illness in the sixties and seventies—think R.D. Laing and psychosis as shamanic journey—and by the inevitable navel gazing that going nuts entails. In *The Eden Express*, Vonnegut writes:

> *Most people assume it must be very painful for me to remember being crazy. It's not true. The fact is, my memories of being crazy give me an almost sensual glee. . . . Everything I did, felt, and said had an awesome grace, symmetry, and perfection to it. . . .*
>
> *It's regrets that make painful memories. When I was crazy I did everything just right.*

In his first memoir, Vonnegut exhibits a rueful self-awareness about the absurdity of his situation. But he still looks back almost lovingly on his psychosis, luxuriating in its drama. In contrast, the voice of his 2010 book feels hacked to the bone:

> *Having a famous parent is a leg up to nowhere. It made sense to people that Kurt Vonnegut's son would have mental health problems. It made sense that I would not do well.*

> *"You're Kurt Vonnegut's son? I heard that you*
> *had hung yourself in a barn in New Jersey."*
> *"No. Actually I'm in med school."*
> *My mother glossed over the chaos we had come*
> *from. "You all turned out so well."*

I don't love *Just Like Someone Without Mental Illness Only More So* the way I did *The Eden Express*, but that makes me trust it more. Like Kurt Vonnegut's fractured stories (a *New York Times* columnist in 1965 dismissed *God Bless You, Mr. Rosewater* as "random meditations" that were "devoid of anything as square as a plot"), Mark Vonnegut's second memoir takes me to unexpected places. With its understated style and sly nod to his father's work, this is the book that really grapples with his regrets.

Stepping off the Eden Express

What *Just Like Someone Without Mental Illness Only More So* offers is a look at the scattered illuminations that drive recovery—not the heroic upward march to mental health, but the wisdom of one who knows that life is tenuous.

Its eighteen short chapters begin with "A Brief Family History" and "Raised by Wolves," which provide the backstory to Vonnegut's mental illness. He describes the many relatives on both sides of his family who suffered from manic depression:

> *We have episodes of hearing voices, delusions,*
> *hyper-religiosity, and periods of not being able to*

> *eat or sleep. These episodes are remarkably similar*
> *across generations and between individuals. It's like*
> *an apocalyptic disintegration sequence that might*
> *be useful if the world really is ending, but if the*
> *world is not ending, you just end up in a nuthouse.*

As a child in the fifties and early sixties, Vonnegut notes, "I was mostly left alone to figure things out." He grew up in a rundown house on Cape Cod, when father Kurt was still trying to make money by selling cars and mother Jane struggled with her own mania.

Young Mark often wandered on his own through woods or even down the shoulder of a four-lane highway with his bicycle. He says that his "proudly antisocial" father—"who spent most of his time at a typewriter, reflecting negatively on his neighbors and society"—considered it a badge of honor his son didn't have any friends.

"I tried to breathe next to no air and leave next to no footprints," Vonnegut writes of his troubled coming of age. But then he adds, deadpan, "A psychotic break is the exact opposite of not taking up much space and being as little trouble as possible."

The book then zips through what happened after he went crazy on the commune, recovered, and wrote *The Eden Express*. Vonnegut attended Harvard Medical School, became a celebrated pediatrician, "cracked up" again in 1985, and then got his life back.

On the surface, it sounds like the usual plotline. The difference comes in Vonnegut's telling the second time around. What could seem meaningful when told as "the story of my life"—the kind of recaps heard in everything from powerhouses like Karr's *Lit* to the average Twelve Step meeting—isn't necessarily meaningful at all.

"Life for the unwell is discontinuous and unpredictable," Vonnegut notes early on. "Things just come out of nowhere. People try but mostly do a lousy job of taking care of you."

Talk about bursting the bubbles of everyone from therapists to literary critics. Those who have been mentally ill all their lives, as my own artist mother was, really are ill. Being crazy isn't a sure ticket to spiritual wisdom or creative transcendence. Vonnegut came to the same conclusion in *The Eden Express*, but it's clear his youthful self had yet to face up to how little he could control his illness.

Now in his sixties, Vonnegut writes that the obvious dramatic elements of his story "do not make a life." But, he concludes with a shrug, "if you add up enough things that aren't in and of themselves enough, it almost starts to add up to something."

Such Kurt Vonnegut-like adages can be annoyingly evasive. The trick, of course, is how you turn a life that's "discontinuous and unpredictable" into a book. *Just Like Someone Without Mental Illness Only More So* is not a page-turner. A third of the way in, I was impatient with its sketchy anecdotes and lack of fully fleshed characters.

Kurt Vonnegut is glimpsed only occasionally: the obsessed writer behind a closed door, simultaneously checked out and too hard on his kids. His death in 2007 (after a fall and head injury) is a denouement of sorts, but a muted one. The passage in which Mark describes acting as his dad's medical proxy—he made sure Kurt wasn't "shipped to a futile neuro-rehab in New Jersey" when nobody else "wanted to be responsible for the death of an icon"—is both profound and too elliptical:

> *So I took care of my father like my father had cut through the crap and taken care of me thirty-six years earlier in British Columbia. I was glad to be able to repay the favor. He took responsibility for hospitalizing me, and I took responsibility for letting him go.*

The terseness of this passage is typical of *Just Like Someone Without Mental Illness Only More So*; Vonnegut resists the urge to dwell in the moment, amplifying its significance. Yet I found myself surprised on every page, asking questions, thinking about whether A connects to B, and realizing, "Ah ha! Maybe they don't."

The Chapter of Revelations

"Crack-up Number Four," the chapter about Vonnegut's psychotic break in 1985, comes at almost the exact midpoint of the book. Suddenly, the more emotionally distanced telling of the first half is wrenched out of joint. This chapter follows a mini-arc, beginning with Vonnegut loving "the rhythm and rank of being a primary-care pediatrician." There's foreboding, then the crash, but the telling is anything but conventional.

The revelation of this chapter comes in its taut little scenes between single asterisks, the descriptions of the voices Vonnegut hears, and what he thought it all meant. His ability to evoke how chronology falls apart during a psychotic episode is masterful.

Many of the "crazy" scenes of *The Eden Express* attempt to do this, too, and they are evocative. But that book's narrative form, with its colorful cast of hippie commune-mates and the linear progression over time, makes even his ravings about iridescent faces and being able to talk to trees seem more orderly than they do in "Crack-up Number Four."

In his second book, Vonnegut describes going crazy as "a grammatical shift. . . . There is no simile or metaphor. There's no tense but the present":

> *It would possibly be tolerable to feel* like *or* as if *one was on fire or* like *the CIA might be after you or* like *you had to hold your breath so that you could be compacted and smuggled to a neutral site in Mongolia to wrestle India's craziest crazy. But there's no* like *or* as if. *It's all really happening, and there's no time to argue or have second thoughts.*

There are wrenching scenes here, sometimes evoked in just a sentence or two. After trying to jump through a third-floor window in his house, Vonnegut was hauled off to the very hospital where he practiced. He describes seeing a nurse whose children he'd treated looking like she wanted to cry: "'Don't worry,' I tried to tell her. 'This will turn out okay.'" Later he reassures his eight-year-old son—"'Things will get better, Zachary'"—knowing that might not be the case.

Vonnegut's version of his experience recognizes the tension that's always present in storytelling—that is, the pull between the random elements of real life and the sense we make of it internally. "All the arts are ways to start a dialogue with yourself," he writes toward the end of the book. That dialogue can be enormously therapeutic, but it's also a faulty and ever-evolving construction.

Finding the Daily Sweetness

"Any way I tell this story is a lie," writes Mary Karr in her prologue to *Lit*, under the title "Open Letter to My Son." This is the brazen approach many readers love her for, and she's right—no well-crafted tale is strictly the truth. The drama is often intensified, as Karr tries to explain here:

> [I]t's a neurological fact that the scared self holds on while the reasoned one lets go. The adrenaline that let our ancestors escape the sabertooth tiger sears into the meat of our brains the extraordinary, the loud. The shrieking fight or the out-of-character insult endures forever, while the daily sweetness dissolves like sugar in water.

Yet Karr's reference to a "neurological fact" that isn't a fact for everyone, as well as phrasing like "sears into the meat of our brains," tips her hand. The drive to tell your own story in a dramatic way always carries a whiff of narcissism. It's all talk, talk, talk, especially in mental-illness and other recovery narratives, which are still strapped by the outmoded belief that the "talking cure"—the awful childhood, the distant father, the drunken mother—can explain the illness.

As literary writers, we're damned if we do and damned if we don't. But I believe it's possible to write in a less melodramatic key.

Just Like Someone Without Mental Illness Only More So captures moments of daily sweetness in the quality of its narrative and in what this author chooses to remember. It reminds me of why I also read literary fiction that resists the rollercoaster ride of the good story, with its overly controlled catharsis and resolution. With both Vonneguts, father and son, the satisfactions come from simple astonishments—the way life is not explained but illuminated.

We all resist the notion that life is a series of scattered moments. Light does occasionally dawn inside our skulls, but then the darkness comes down again. My mother on her worst days wanted it all to mean something. In both his memoirs, Mark Vonnegut calls "too much meaning" one of the chief problems of psychosis. The craziness makes everything appear connected and intentional, from God to John Coltrane to the goats on the farm—with paranoia as one of the most florid forms of storytelling.

There's a plot, all right. But it means far less than the realization that nobody is actually in charge or working the levers of the universe.

In the 2002 reissue of *The Eden Express*, a new foreword by Kurt Vonnegut brings back his remarkable voice and existential attitude so clearly I want to quote the whole thing, and I encourage readers to look it up. Here, I'll settle for one passage. Of the dire days when his son was admitted to a "Canuck loony bin," he wrote:

> And I recall now a time when I pondered buying from a gift shop a pretty object sacred to believers in a faith I knew nothing about. Only kidding, I asked the woman who waited on me if she thought it would bring me bad luck if I treated it disrespectfully. Only kidding, she replied, "That depends, I would think, on how many hostages you have given to fortune."
>
> I found her answer so unexpectedly eloquent and poignant that I supposed it to be a quotation. I have since looked it up. It was written by Francis Bacon, and reads in full: "He that hath wife and children hath given hostages to fortune."
>
> Indeed, indeed!

"I've found it helps a lot to get older," Mark Vonnegut says in his second book. It's a small epiphany, neither loud nor extraordinary, and I'm grateful for it. He adds, "Now when honking cars start sounding like my name or other things happen that could be the voices warming up, I'm not thrilled or terrified. 'I've got a lot going on,' I say. 'You'll have to wait your turn.'"

Sources

Just Like Someone Without Mental Illness Only More So: A Memoir by Mark Vonnegut (Delacorte/Random House, 2010).

The Eden Express: A Memoir of Insanity by Mark Vonnegut, originally published by Praeger Publishers in 1975 (Seven Stories Press, 2002).

"Just Like Someone Without Mental Illness Only More So: A Memoir," review by *Publisher's Weekly*, May 31, 2010.

Quote about *God Bless You, Mr. Rosewater* is from "Do Human Beings Matter?" by Martin Levin, *New York Times*, April 25, 1965.

Lit: A Memoir by Mary Karr (HarperCollins, 2009).

CONTRIBUTORS' NOTES

Martha Nichols is the Editor-in-Chief of *Talking Writing*, a nonprofit digital magazine, and the editor of *Into Sanity*. She is also a faculty instructor in journalism at the Harvard University Extension School. Her nonfiction has appeared in *Salon*, *Women's Review of Books*, *Utne Reader*, and *Christian Science Monitor*, among others. She's especially interested in first-person journalism.

Mark Vonnegut is the author of *The Eden Express* and *Just Like Someone Without Mental Illness Only More So*.

Jane McCafferty writes fiction, nonfiction, and poetry. She is the author of two novels (HarperCollins) and two books of short stories (HarperCollins and University of Pittsburgh Press, later reissued by Carnegie Mellon Press). Her work has received many awards, including an NEA, the Pushcart Prize for both fiction and essay, the Drue Heinz Award, a Book Sense award, and the Great Lakes New Writers Award. She teaches a variety of writing courses at Carnegie Mellon University and is cofounder of the Pittsburgh Memoir project, for which she facilitates writing workshops for people in the community.

> ➤ *Jane McCafferty won the 2016 Talking Writing Prize for Personal Essay.*

Beth Richards is a north Florida native who lives and works in Connecticut. Her work has appeared in *Fourth Genre*; *Solstice Literary Magazine: A Magazine of Diverse Voices*; and the anthology *Crooked Letter i: Coming out in the South.* She is a graduate of the Solstice MFA in Creative Writing Program at Pine Manor College and directs the first- and second-year writing programs at the University of Hartford. This essay is part of a memoir in progress.

Sara Hubbs is a multimedia artist and writer originally from Phoenix, Arizona. She completed an MFA in Visual Art at the George Washington University in Washington, D.C., and has shown nationally and internationally in Mexico City, Abu Dhabi, New York City, and elsewhere. Sara's prose work was chosen for the 2017 Tucson Festival of Books Masters Workshop. She lives in Tucson with her husband and daughter.

Greg Correll was a 2017 fellow at the CUNY Graduate Center's Writers Institute, where he worked closely with Leo Carey (*New Yorker*) and Jonathan Galassi (Farrar, Straus & Giroux). He wrote about his Parkinson's diagnosis for *Salon* and about sexual assaults in jail as a fourteen-year-old for the *Good*

Men Project. He's been published in half a dozen essay and poetry anthologies, and two of his short plays have been produced, one of them off-Broadway. He's channeled his PTSD hypomania into art—he won a CLIO for package design and illustrated for the *New Yorker*—and science—he engineered the Yale Climate Institute's scientific collaboration system/site. He also works as a freelance editor and loves helping writers improve and polish their work.

Rae Alexandra Underberg graduated from Georgetown University with a BA in English and Psychology. She is currently a case manager at a Brooklyn nonprofit, working on alternatives to incarceration and detention.

Kristine Snow Millard began her writing career in 1985 as a newspaper reporter in Gloucester, Massachusetts. After a detour to law school and a legal career, she resumed writing in the late 1990s. She earned an MFA in creative nonfiction from the University of Southern Maine's Stonecoast Program in Creative Writing in 2016. She is currently writing a memoir about the impact—and unexpected lessons—of living with mental illness. Kristine lives with her husband in Saco, Maine. They have two grown daughters.

Lorri McDole is a writer who lives with her family in the Pacific Northwest. Her writing has appeared in publications that include *The Writer, Cleaver, Sweet, The Offing, Essay Daily, New*

Madrid, and *Brain, Child*. She has also been published in several anthologies and been a finalist in several contests. She is currently working on a flash nonfiction chapbook.

    ◆ *Lorri McDole was a finalist for the 2016 Talking Writing Prize for Personal Essay.*

Amy McVay Abbott is a retired health-care executive who lives in Indiana with her husband, Randy. She is one of forty women featured in the first anthology published by the Erma Bombeck Writer's Workshop: *Laugh Out Loud: 40 Female Humorists Celebrate Then and Now, Before We Forget* (University of Dayton, 2018). Abbott, who is syndicated on Senior Wire News Service, writes about health, the arts, travel, humor, and politics in print and online, and is the author of four books.

Madeleine Holman was born in New York and grew up in Paris, London, Tokyo, and Connecticut. She was an early member of the Austin, Texas, affiliate of the National Alliance on Mental Illness and the group's president for two years. She lives with her husband in Austin, where she writes, paints, and draws. "What If" is adapted from a longer essay and a memoir-in-progress.

Drew Ciccolo has had short stories published in *The Masters Review* and *Tin House*. "Paige," his lone work of nonfiction to date, came out of a course he took in the Rutgers-Newark MFA program with Alice Elliott Dark in the fall of 2012. The year prior, he had experienced the deaths of his mother and younger sister within six months of each other.

> ❧ *Drew Ciccolo won the 2013 Talking Writing Prize for Creative Nonfiction.*

Joanna Brichetto is a naturalist in Nashville, Tennessee, the hackberry capital of the world. She writes the urban nature blog *Look Around: Nearby Nature*, and her essays have appeared in *Hippocampus*, *The Hopper*, *Flyway*, *storySouth*, *The Common*, *About Place Journal*, *City Creatures Blog*, *Longleaf Review*, *The Fourth River*, and other journals.

Carl Bowlby lives in the Berkshires of western Massachusetts with his daughter. He has been writing his entire life, although he can claim only one other publishing credit to his name: a poem called "Hot Wind Someday" in the Irish literary journal *The Moth* (Winter 2014-15). Carl is extremely pleased this piece has been chosen for inclusion in *Talking Writing*'s anthology on mental illness—a personal concern for him.

Linda Saslow is a reading tutor who lives in Fullerton, California, with her husband. She thanks Dana Goodyear of the *New Yorker* for advising her on the first draft of this essay, which was included in Linda's thesis for her master's degree in professional writing at the University of Southern California. She also thanks numerous graduates of the USC program who meet regularly as part of Sunday Writers Unblocked for input on crafting this essay.

Kim Triedman is an award-winning poet, novelist, and visual artist. She's had three poetry collections published as well as her 2013 novel, *The Other Room*. She lives in the Boston area.

Marianne Goldsmith is the pen name of Marianne Smith, a San Francisco Bay Area resident for more than thirty years. She studied literature at Pitzer College in California and in France, and holds an MA in Creative Writing from San Francisco State University. She works as a writer, editor, and communications professional. She is also a political activist and education advocate. Her work has appeared in *Poetry Flash*, *SF Bay Guardian*, *Persimmon Tree*, and the anthology *Times They Were A-Changing: Women Remember the '60s and '70s (*She Writes Press, 2013*)*.

Rebecca Schumejda is the author of several full-length poetry collections, including *Falling Forward* (Sunny Outside Press, 2009), *Cadillac Men* (NYQ Books, 2013), *Waiting at the Dead End Diner* (Bottom Dog Press, 2014), *Our One-Way Street* NYQ Books, 2017), and several chapbooks. She graduated with her master's in creative writing and poetics from San Francisco State University. She currently lives in New York's Hudson Valley with her family. Schumejda is working on a collection that addresses mental illness, tragedy, and incarceration. Some of those pieces have been published in *Borderlands Texas Poetry Review*, *Cape Rock*, *Gravel*, *Juked*, *Main Street Rag*, *Open Minds Quarterly*, and the *Pikeville Review*.

Julie Evans is a licensed massage therapist, an ordained deacon, and a freelance writer. In addition to her regular column for *Healthy You* magazine, Julie has been published in the *Woodstock Times, Healthy Hudson Valley, Pulse* magazine, *Fictionique,* and NPR's *The Roundtable.* She has also written a memoir, *Joy Road: My Journey from Addiction to Recovery* (Woodstock Arts, 2019). Julie believes that words and touch are among our best medicines.

April Newman is a professor and writer. Her work has appeared in the *Iowa Review, Mindful Metropolis, Hypertext,* and the anthology *Windy City Queer: LGBTQ Dispatches from the Third Coast* (University of Wisconsin Press, 2011). Her writing has been recognized in *New Millennium Writings* and by Columbia University's Scholastic Press Association. She lives in Chicago with her wife, Kara, and French bulldog, Hugo.

Joe Vastano started writing at sixteen. He traced Jim Morrison to Kerouac and Rimbaud, took them at their words, and deranged his senses on the road for twenty years. Now, he's sorting through it all.

Maureen Sullivan received her MFA in creative writing from Pacific University in 2015. She's had an essay published in *Wildbranch: An Anthology of Nature, Environmental, and Place-based Writing.* She is working on a memoir about the reverberations of her childhood in the Yankee state of Pennsylvania with a crazy Southern mother. Reckoning with her Southern bloodline has flummoxed her more than accepting her mother's mental illness. Maureen lives in the Pacific Northwest with her husband, daughter, two large dogs, and, in the good years, a few hundred-thousand Italian honeybees.

Jamie Passaro is a writer who runs the *Dear Person* website for obituaries (dearpersonobits.com). Her articles, interviews, and essays have been published in the *New York Times*, the *Washington Post*, the *Atlantic*, *Full Grown People*, the *Sun*, *Utne Reader*, and *Oregon Humanities Magazine*, among other places. She lives in Eugene, Oregon, with her husband and two daughters.

We hope you enjoyed this book. Would you do us a favor?

Like all authors, we at Talking Writing Books rely on online reviews to encourage future sales. Your opinion is invaluable. Would you take a few moments now to share your assessment of this anthology on Amazon or any other book-review website you prefer? Your opinion will help the book marketplace become more transparent and useful to all.

Thank you very much!

ABOUT TALKING WRITING

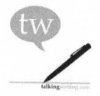

TW: literature + journalism

Talking Writing is a nonprofit literary site that features essays, first-person journalism, visual art, fiction, and poetry. Our mission? To show why writing matters in the digital age—and why good reporting and storytelling can change the world.

Since its founding in 2010 as an independent 501(c)(3) charitable organization, *Talking Writing* has produced a wealth of material by diverse authors. Talking Writing Books brings their words to print, featuring anthologies of TW's best work.

CPSIA information can be obtained
at www.ICGtesting.com
Printed in the USA
LVHW091759201119
638021LV00002B/208/P